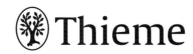

Surgery for Rheumatic Diseases

Stefan Sell, MD, PhD
Professor
Medical Director
Center for Joint Surgery
Enzkreiskliniken Neuenbürg
Neuenbürg, Germany

Stefan Rehart, MD, PhD
Professor
Director Department of Orthopaedics and Trauma Surgery
Agaplesion Markus Hospital
Agaplesion Frankfurter Diakonie Health Group gGmbH
Frankfurt, Germany

434 illustrations

Thieme
Stuttgart • New York • Delhi • Rio de Janeiro

Library of Congress Cataloging-in-Publication Data is available from the publisher.

This book is an authorized translation of the first German edition published and copyrighted 2013 by Georg Thieme Verlag, Stuttgart. Title of the German edition: Operationsatlas Orthopädische Rheumatologie.

Translator: Cornelia Riedl, Milwaukee, WI, USA
Illustrator: Malgorzata & Piotr Gusta, Paris, France

© 2017 Georg Thieme Verlag KG

Thieme Publishers Stuttgart
Rüdigerstrasse 14, 70469 Stuttgart, Germany
+49 [0]711 8931 421, customerservice@thieme.de

Thieme Publishers New York
333 Seventh Avenue, New York, NY 10001 USA
+1 800 782 3488, customerservice@thieme.com

Thieme Publishers Delhi
A-12, Second Floor, Sector-2, Noida-201301
Uttar Pradesh, India
+91 120 45 566 00, customerservice@thieme.in

Thieme Publishers Rio de Janeiro, Thieme Publicações Ltda.
Edifício Rodolpho de Paoli, 25º andar
Av. Nilo Peçanha, 50 – Sala 2508
Rio de Janeiro 20020-906 Brasil
+55 21 3172 2297 / +55 21 3172 1896

Cover design: Thieme Publishing Group
Typesetting by DiTech Process Solutions Pvt. Ltd., India

Printed in China by Everbest Printing Ltd., Hong Kong   5 4 3 2 1

ISBN 978-3-13-240007-8

Also available as an e-book:
eISBN 978-3-13-241449-5

Contents

Preface

What makes surgery on rheumatoid patients so different?

Our goal was to draw on our 25 years of experience in this specialty to present our perspective of the operative management of rheumatoid patients. This atlas is aimed at experienced surgeons interested in rheumatic orthopaedics and also orthopaedic and trauma surgeons who wish to learn more about orthopaedic rheumatology. The intention was not to illustrate every single aspect of rheumatic orthopaedics but rather to give an overview of standard surgical procedures.

After a busy day in the operating room followed by a mountain of administrative tasks, we, like our colleagues, often found it difficult to spend our evenings reading textbooks in preparation for the following day's surgical procedures. Most of the time, we would fall asleep before reaching the end of a chapter. Because of this, our aim was to present our ideas on planning surgical procedures in a very visual way, and so the text plays only a secondary role. This approach is particularly suitable for our colleagues in surgery, many of whom are often extremely visually oriented, and may find it easier to integrate the knowledge gained this way into their surgical practice. There is a much higher chance that a tired orthopaedic or trauma surgeon will be able to spend an evening reading well-illustrated surgical chapters and stay awake while doing so.

At the same time, we hope to share with our younger colleagues some of our own enthusiasm for rheumatic orthopaedics.

Professor Stefan Sell, MD, PhD
Professor Stefan Rehart, MD, PhD

Contributors

Heinrich Boehm, MD
Associate Professor
Director Department of Spine Surgery
Bad Berka Medical Center
Bad Berka, Germany

Christof Chan, MD
Nagold, Germany

Vladimir Crnic, MD
Department of Endoprosthetics and Joint Surgery
Center for Degenerative Joint and Rheumatic Diseases
Bad Wildbad, Germany

Martina Henniger, MD
Department of Orthopaedics and Trauma Surgery
Agaplesion Markus Hospital
Agaplesion Frankfurter Diakonie Health Group gGmbH
Frankfurt, Germany

Boris Kurosch, MD
Stuttgart, Germany

Angela Lehr
Department of Orthopaedics and Trauma Surgery
Agaplesion Markus Hospital
Agaplesion Frankfurter Diakonie Health Group gGmbH
Frankfurt, Germany

Axel Lust
Department of Orthopaedics and Trauma Surgery
Agaplesion Markus Hospital

Agaplesion Frankfurter Diakonie Health Group gGmbH
Frankfurt, Germany

Stefan Rehart, MD, PhD
Professor
Director Department of Orthopaedics and Trauma Surgery
Agaplesion Markus Hospital
Agaplesion Frankfurter Diakonie Health Group gGmbH
Frankfurt, Germany

Joerg Richard, MD
Herxheim, Germany

Alexandra Sachs
Department of Orthopaedics and Trauma Surgery
Agaplesion Markus Hospital
Agaplesion Frankfurter Diakonie Health Group gGmbH
Frankfurt, Germany

Alexander Schoeniger
Department of Orthopaedics and Trauma Surgery
Agaplesion Markus Hospital
Agaplesion Frankfurter Diakonie Health Group gGmbH
Frankfurt, Germany

Stefan Sell, MD, PhD
Professor
Medical Director
Center for Joint Surgery
Enzkreiskliniken Neuenbürg
Neuenbürg, Germany

Chapter 1

Principles of Orthopaedic Rheumatology

1 Principles of Orthopaedic Rheumatology

S. Sell, S. Rehart

Rheumatoid arthritis is a chronic systemic inflammatory autoimmune disorder that can progress to involve all of the synovial tissues and even the internal organs. The inflammatory reaction begins in the joints and can lead to irreversible damage. Depending on the acuteness of the situation, either a rheumatologist or an orthopaedic surgeon assumes responsibility for management of disease progression when patients require treatment. A combination of physical therapy, occupational therapy, medical social services, orthopaedic technology, and psychological care is utilized in a multidisciplinary approach. Patient support associations (for example, the European League Against Rheumatism [EULAR]) and other specialties also provide assistance.

Joint swelling with effusions and synovitis are characteristic of rheumatoid disease. If left untreated for more than 6 weeks, the inflammation can cause joint damage with deformities and dislocations. A similar process leads to tenosynovitis and can also affect the visceral organs. Early confirmation of the diagnosis (EULAR classification criteria) is based on clinical signs and laboratory results.

Medical drug therapy is imperative. A rheumatologist typically makes the initial and differential diagnoses and initiates appropriate antirheumatic drug therapy. Oral administration of glucocorticoid medication often leads to a rapid relief of symptoms. However, long-term control or even remission requires administration of DMARDs (disease-modifying antirheumatic drugs). Methotrexate is the gold standard and modern biologicals are frequently added as immunomodulators, either in combination or as an alternative treatment.

Preoperatively, particular attention should be given to the risks of impaired wound healing, infection, and thrombosis. These risks are already elevated due to the underlying illness and may be potentiated by medication therapy. Perioperative management of antirheumatic medications is based on the extent of the surgical procedure, the age of the patient, the amount of disease activity, and other comorbidities. The perioperative medication management plan should be discussed with the patient and coordinated with the treating rheumatologist. Recommendations for management of biologic agents have been developed by the German Society for Rheumatology (Deutsche Gesellschaft für Rheumatologie [DGRh]).

We discontinue biologicals perioperatively. The increased risk of a drug-related postoperative infection is weighed against the possibility that an interruption of immunosuppressive therapy could trigger another serious flare in the underlying illness. There is no standardized approach and definitive studies are not yet available. Care must be taken to discontinue biologic immunosuppressive medication at least 2 half-lives prior to surgery. A washout procedure with cholestyramine is usually advisable when discontinuing leflunomide because of its high degree of tissue binding.

For patients taking glucocorticoids at doses high enough to cause Cushing's syndrome, a perioperative cortisone regimen (based on the extent of the surgical intervention) is recommended for prophylaxis against an Addisonian crisis.

Immunosuppressive medications can be resumed once the wound has completely healed.

The type of surgical intervention is typically dictated by the stage of the disease. In the early stages with joint swelling that persists despite optimization of oral medication therapy and intra-articular cortisone injections, the initial surgical treatment is arthroscopy and synovectomy. To help prevent recurrence, synovectomies are usually combined with radiosynoviorthesis 6 weeks postoperatively.

More advanced findings such as bone and cartilage destruction (Larsen > III) may require prosthetic implants, arthroplasties, and arthrodesis.

We find it important not to miss appropriate timing for surgical interventions. Reconstructive procedures may slow disease progression, particularly in the hands and feet. Thus, for example, radiolunate arthrodesis is recommended for an unstable wrist (Schulthess classification) in order to counteract subluxation. The same applies to the foot: osteotomies are a good option if the joints have not yet been destroyed and the soft tissues can still be reconstructed.

Because "rheumatic" patients require a large number of surgical interventions and hospital stays, a patient-oriented treatment approach should be considered. It is preferable to begin with the "best surgical procedure," that is, one that will provide the patient with a rapid and sustained improvement in symptoms. In addition, patients should be given an expected timeframe for recovery: for example, when they can resume walking or when they can return to work.

To preserve mobility in patients with severe and simultaneous involvement of both upper and lower extremities, surgical treatment of the lower extremity is crucial. It is also reasonable to perform combined complex hand and foot operations; alternatively, several procedures can be performed simultaneously on multiple small joints/tendons located on a single extremity. In individual cases simultaneous bilateral operations can be performed on the lower extremities. These include total hip arthroplasty, total knee arthroplasty, and complex forefoot procedures.

Furthermore, the rule "proximal before distal" applies.

Preoperative evaluation of "rheumatic patients" includes a general physical examination, blood sampling, a detailed discussion with the surgeon, and an anesthesiology assessment with particular focus on temporomandibular joint function and cervical spine mobility. Radiographic imaging of the specific joint to be operated on and functional imaging of the cervical spine (lateral view of cervical spine with head in flexion, centered on C1, and hard palate) to exclude C1–C2 subluxation should also be performed.

Postoperatively, early physiotherapeutic mobilization is particularly important in patients with chronic inflammatory joint diseases. This often requires special aids adapted to the individual patient (e.g., underarm crutches with ergonomic handles, forearm supports, or armpit supports). Optimal postoperative care should include early occupational therapy and use of orthopaedic aids.

Chapter 2

The Hand

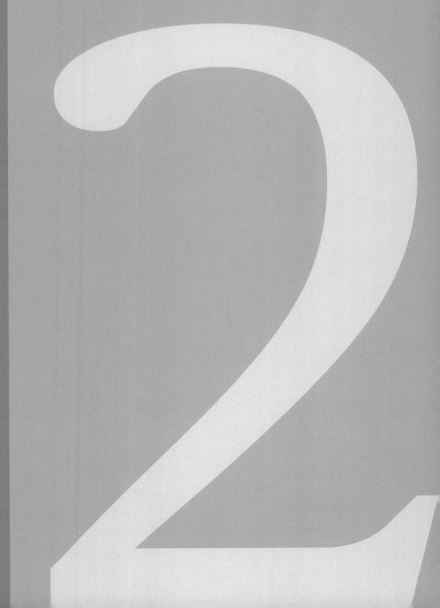

2 The Hand

S. Rehart, S. Sell, B. Kurosch, J. Richard

2.1 General

The assessment of treatment indications for the rheumatic hand is easily one of the most difficult topics in orthopaedic rheumatology.

Determining an optimal course of treatment for the patient requires simultaneous consideration of many factors. The hand's current functional limitations need to be evaluated within the context of the underlying destruction and dysfunction of the hand structures, as well as the patient's overall disease-related limitations. An in-depth knowledge of the different courses of specific rheumatic illness is essential for determining an indication for treatment. For example, does the patient have psoriatic arthritis that is more prone to ankyloses, or destabilizing arthritis that leads to instability?

The level of destruction plays only a limited role in determining the extent of surgical intervention. The best functional improvement is achieved by arthrodesis of the thumb carpometacarpal joint. Consequently, this type of intervention paves the way for and creates the necessary confidence in additional and potentially more major procedures. For it to be possible to give patients a timeline for surgical improvement of their hand, a therapeutic plan is often essential:

- Stabilization of the wrist joint.
- Swanson prosthesis of the metacarpophalangeal (MCP) joint.
- Arthrodesis of the proximal interphalangeal (PIP) joint.

The importance of functional aftercare must be discussed with the patient from the outset because it is one of the keys to success.

It is relatively easy to determine indications for treatment of the hand in urgent or emergent situations. First and foremost among these are tendon ruptures. However, even these can be tolerated by some patients for months or years. The goal is to treat flexor or extensor tendon ruptures as quickly as possible. From both technical and functional standpoints, the more time that elapses after the initial event, the more difficult treatment of these ruptures becomes.

An end-to-end suture repair is only rarely feasible because the tissue is usually too damaged and the tendons have retracted too far. Side-to-side repair is possible for extensive ruptures, and a free transplant (for example, using the palmaris longus tendon) is an option for large defects. In these situations functional aftercare and, ultimately, outcomes are clearly more challenging.

A rupture of the tendon of the extensor pollicis longus (EPL) muscle, the most common tendon rupture of the hand, represents a special situation. It typically involves performing a surgical transposition of the tendon of the extensor indicis proprius muscle, although this requires lengthy follow-up treatment. Arthrodesis of the interphalangeal joint of the thumb presents an alternative and should be considered depending upon the amount of hand involvement and level of overall disease. Functionality should also be discussed with the patient.

The indications are much more obvious if there is medial nerve compression accompanied by significant inflammatory symptoms. Here patients usually seek medical care themselves due to pain. In addition to decompression of the median nerve, it is crucial to perform an extensive synovectomy of the flexor tendons.

Treatment indications for tenosynovitis, in contrast, are often more difficult to recognize and not as easy for patients to accept. Here the swelling in the hand is painless and, as long as tendon rupture has not occurred, does not impair the patient.

As a general rule for surgical correction of the hand: Start proximal, move distal!

For example, a soft tissue repair of an ulnar deviation of the MCP joint seems futile if the wrist has a severe axial deviation located more proximally. The repair inevitably results in recurrence.

According to the Schulthess classification of rheumatic wrist disease, there are three different progressive forms:

- Arthritic.
- Ankylosing.
- Destabilizing.

The destabilizing progressive form, which leads to ulnar dislocation, usually originates from scapholunate (SL) ligament disruption. It must be recognized early in order to perform a radiolunate arthrodesis as this type of arthrodesis requires an intact distal wrist joint.

It is often difficult to determine indications for soft tissue repairs on MCP joints or swan neck/boutonnière deformities. There cannot be too much bone damage and the soft tissues must still be amenable to repair through a release. At the same time, there must still be sufficient long-term stability of the soft tissues after they are surgically repaired or transposed. Accurate assessment requires many years of experience treating rheumatic hands.

Clearly, it is much harder to determine the correct treatment indications than to perform the operative intervention itself.

2.2 The Wrist

2.2.1 Arthroscopic Synovectomy of the Wrist

▶ **Indication.** Therapy resistant Larsen 0–II/III synovitis after optimization of medication therapy and cortisone injections.

Extensor tendon synovitis, which is frequently present, requires an open procedure.

▶ **Specific disclosures for patient consent.** Recurrence. Infection. Radiosynoviorthesis or chemosynoviorthesis may be necessary 6 weeks postoperatively.

▶ **Instruments.** Standard small joint arthroscope. Camera. Shaver system. Electrocautery.

▶ **Position.** Supine. Tourniquet on the proximal upper arm. The arm is suspended using a wrist traction device with the elbow joint in 90° of flexion. The suspension device is draped in a sterile fashion (▶ Fig. 2.2). Weights (ca. 3 kg each) are hung on both sides.

▶ **Approach.** See ▶ Fig. 2.1.

▶ **Specifics.** See ▶ Fig. 2.3, ▶ Fig. 2.4, ▶ Fig. 2.5, ▶ Fig. 2.6. Prior to insertion of the trocar, the radiocarpal joint is insufflated through the 3/4 (radiocarpal) portal using a syringe. The probe and shaver are initially inserted through the 4/5 portal, and then later switched. Finally, the midcarpal joint is accessed via the midcarpal radial (MCR) and midcarpal ulnar (MCU) portals.

▶ **Key steps.** Arthroscopy should be performed carefully in the small spaces to avoid iatrogenic cartilage injuries.

▶ **Operative technique.** See ▶ Fig. 2.7, ▶ Fig. 2.8.

▶ **Specific complications.** Recurrence. Progression of destruction. Development of a supination deformity.

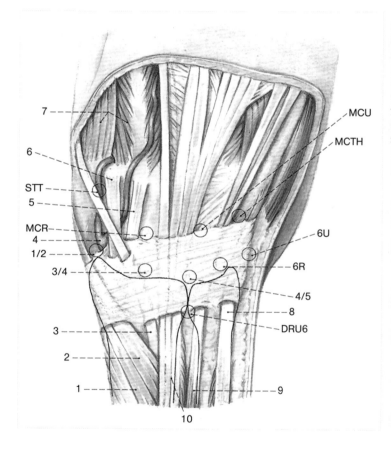

Fig. 2.1 Anatomical view of the arthroscopic portals. 1, Abductor pollicis longus muscle. 2, Extensor pollicis brevis muscle. 3, EPL muscle. 4, Radial artery in the snuff box (tabatière). 5, Extensor carpi radialis longus muscle. 6, Extensor carpi radialis brevis muscle. 7, First dorsal interosseous muscle. 8, Extensor carpi ulnaris muscle. 9, Extensor digiti minimi muscle. 10, Extensor digitorum muscle. STT, os scaphoideum, trapezium, trapezoideum. DRU, distal radioulnar joint. (From Kremer K, Lierse W, Platzer W, Schreiber HW, Weller S. Chirurgische Operationslehre Arthroskopie – obere und untere Extremität. Stuttgart: Thieme; 1997.)

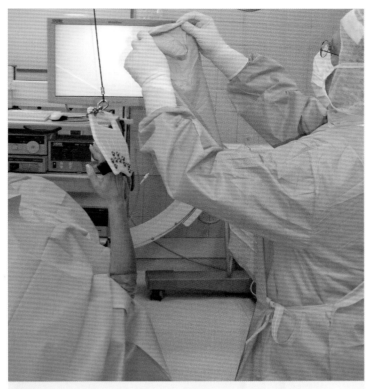

Fig. 2.2 The wrist traction device is draped in a sterile fashion.

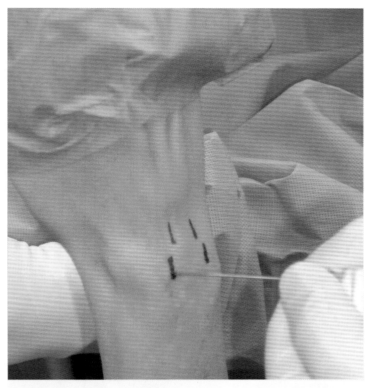

Fig. 2.3 The 3/4 and 4/5 radiocarpal and the midcarpal (MCR and MCU) portals are marked after palpation. The joint is punctured and insufflated with a syringe. Synovial fluid is withdrawn for analysis, if needed.

Fig. 2.4 A miniature camera is inserted into the radial 3/4 portal.

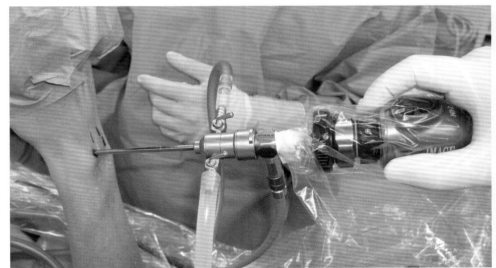

Fig. 2.5 View of an ulnar triangular fibro-cartilage complex (TFCC) lesion with severe synovitis.

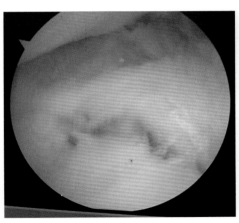

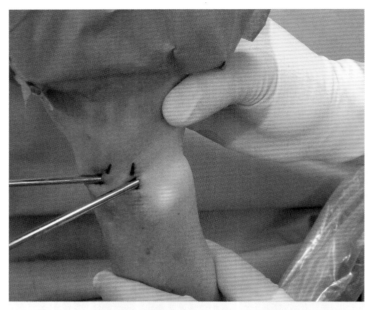

Fig. 2.6 A second portal (4/5) is placed under direct visualization and instruments are inserted (here a shaver).

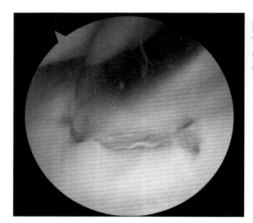

Fig. 2.7 The frayed TFCC is shaved and a synovectomy is performed.

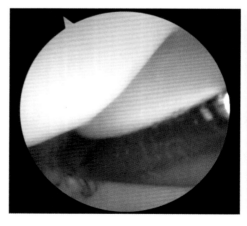

Fig. 2.8 Midcarpal synovitis is evident and is removed by a palmar synovectomy using the shaver (view of the joint between the hamate and capitate).

2.2.2 Radiolunate Arthrodesis

▶ **Indication.** Larsen III–IV destruction with significant clinical symptoms. Radiocarpal joint supination deformity with ulnar drift and palmar subluxation. Radiologically progressive destabilizing form. Impending extensor tendon rupture.

Note that there should be no more than moderate midcarpal destruction.

Consider performing a radioscapholunate arthrodesis if there is pronounced radioscaphoid joint destruction. A Mannerfelt arthrodesis or a prosthesis is indicated for midcarpal destruction.

▶ **Specific disclosures for patient consent.** Loosening, breakage, or dislocation of staples. Tendon rupture (also secondary). Perioperative impact on flexor tendons and median nerve. Loss of wrist function. Pseudarthrosis. Bone fracture/perforation. Damage to sensory cutaneous nerve branches. Resection of the ipsilateral ulnar head is often necessary and cancellous bone is harvested to place into the radiolunate (RL) arthrodesis site.

▶ **Instruments.** Stapler with 10 × 15-mm or 16 × 15-mm staples. Standard hand surgery set.

▶ **Position.** Supine. Hand table. Arrange for perioperative mobile radiography.

▶ **Approach.** See ▶ Fig. 2.9.

▶ **Specifics.** Preoperatively, fit a palmar plaster splint that is to be applied immediately postoperatively.

A residual midcarpal range of motion of 30°–0°–30° extension–flexion can be expected postoperatively.

▶ **Key steps.** Precisely match the resection surfaces of the distal radius lunate fossa and the decorticated proximal lunate surfaces. Firmly reduce and hold the surfaces together during staple insertion. Resect the interosseous branch of the radial nerve on the floor of the fourth extensor tendon compartment.

▶ **Surgical technique.** See ▶ Fig. 2.10, ▶ Fig. 2.11, ▶ Fig. 2.12, ▶ Fig. 2.13, ▶ Fig. 2.14, ▶ Fig. 2.15, ▶ Fig. 2.16, ▶ Fig. 2.17, ▶ Fig. 2.18, ▶ Fig. 2.19.

▶ **Specific complications.** Fracture and dislocation of staples. Pseudarthrosis (often asymptomatic).

▶ **Postoperative aftercare.** Radiographic imaging at 2 and 6 weeks postoperatively.

Immobilization in the plaster splint (palmar plaster splint, with fingers freely mobile at the MCP joints) until stitches are removed 14 days postoperatively. Then an additional 2 to 4 weeks of immobilization in a forearm circular cast. Cast removal is dependent upon follow-up radiographic findings. See ▶ Fig. 2.20 for an 8-year follow-up.

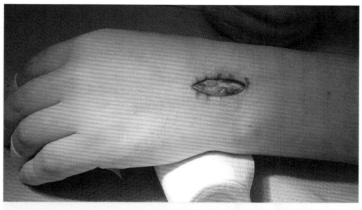

Fig. 2.9 A longitudinal midline incision of ca. 4 cm is made dorsal to the fourth extensor tendon compartment. An oblique approach is an alternative.

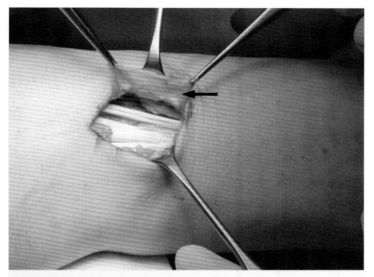

Fig. 2.10 View of the fourth extensor tendon compartment after dividing the extensor retinaculum (arrow).

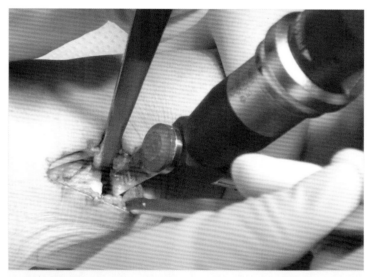

Fig. 2.11 The ulnar head capsule is opened longitudinally. A synovectomy is performed in both pronated and supinated position. For ulnar head destruction, the ulnar head is sparingly resected using the oscillating saw (see also Chapter 2.2.3).

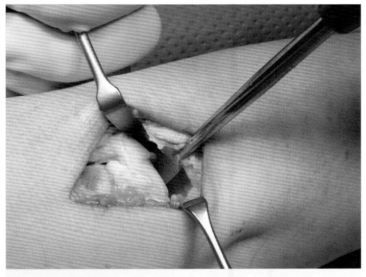

Fig. 2.12 The wrist joint is opened with a V-shaped capsulotomy. The radiolunate joint is mobilized and inspected to evaluate the condition of the cartilage.

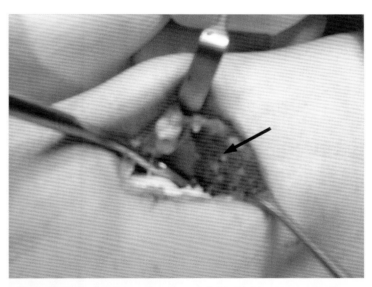

Fig. 2.13 The resection surfaces are debrided with a Luer and a Lexer chisel (with the aid of an awl or a K-wire). Articular surface with cartilage excised (arrow).

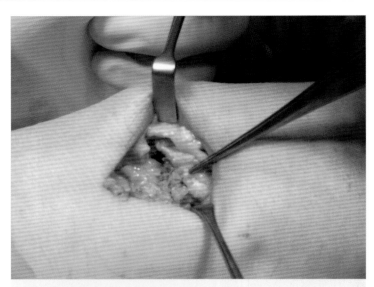

Fig. 2.14 The lunate bone is repositioned dorsally and radially over the radius. Temporary K-wire fixation is used if necessary.

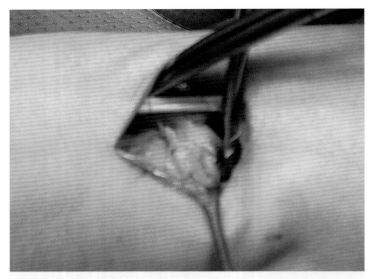

Fig. 2.15 Cancellous bone (derived mainly from the resected ulnar head) is placed after the lunate bone has been reduced.

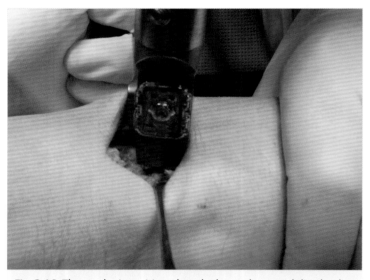

Fig. 2.16 The stapler is positioned on the lunate bone and distal radius and staples are inserted.

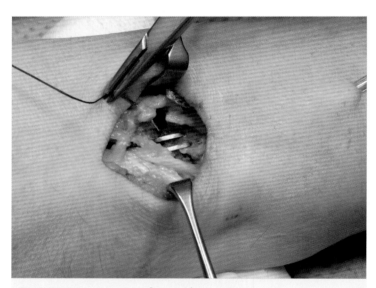

Fig. 2.17 Operative view after staple insertion.

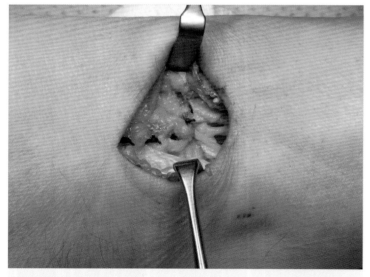

Fig. 2.18 The joint capsule is closed meticulously. In a rheumatoid joint with a thinned capsule, the extensor retinaculum is horizontally split and one half is sutured to the capsule as reinforcement.

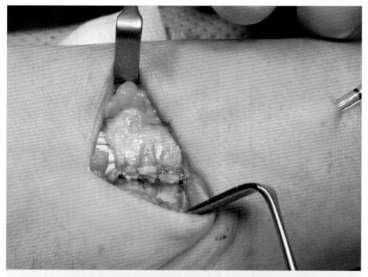

Fig. 2.19 The tendons are then repositioned and the extensor retinaculum is reconstructed.

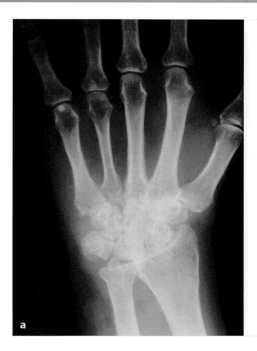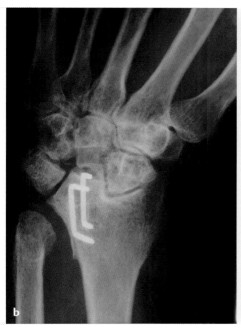

Fig. 2.20 (a,b) Eight-year follow-up after radiolunate arthrodesis. Wrist destabilization has not progressed.

2.2.3 Ulnar Head Resection

▶ **Indication.** Larsen II–III destruction of the radioulnar joint with instability and pain that limits forearm rotational movement. Synovitis. (Pseudo-)Prominence of the ulnar head with skin breakdown imminent or impending rupture of the fourth or fifth digit extensor tendons.

▶ **Specific disclosures for patient consent.** Wrist joint extension/flexion range of motion may be reduced by as much as 30%. Reduced distal radioulnar joint (DRUJ) range of motion for pronation and supination.

▶ **Instruments.** Standard hand surgery set. Oscillating saw.

▶ **Position.** Supine. Hand table.

▶ **Specifics.** A tenosynovectomy of the entire wrist and extensor tendons is also typically performed. Ulnar head resection is frequently combined with a partial radiocarpal arthrodesis

(radiolunate or radioscapholunate) due to anticipated instability. Alternatively, a split tendon transfer using the extensor carpi radialis brevis (ECRB) tendon or a Sauvé–Kapandji procedure (distal ulnar segment resection and radioulnar fusion) can be performed.

▶ **Approach.** A dorsal longitudinal incision is made over the wrist and continued over the DRUJ. A lateral incision over the distal end of the ulna is used only for isolated ulnar head resection. See ▶ Fig. 2.21, ▶ Fig. 2.22, ▶ Fig. 2.23.

▶ **Key steps.** Meticulous joint tenosynovectomy, capsule reconstruction, and repositioning of the extensor carpi ulnaris muscle tendon over the ulnar head.

▶ **Surgical technique.** See ▶ Fig. 2.24, ▶ Fig. 2.25, ▶ Fig. 2.26, ▶ Fig. 2.27, ▶ Fig. 2.28.

▶ **Specific complications.** Progressive ulnar translocation of the carpus may occur if only an isolated ulnar head resection is performed without carpal fixation.

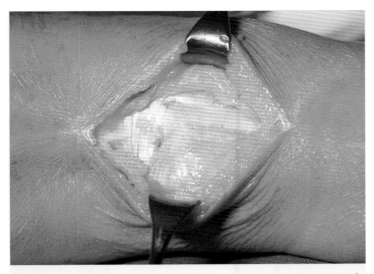

Fig. 2.21 A dorsal longitudinal skin incision is made over the DRUJ and the extensor retinaculum is exposed.

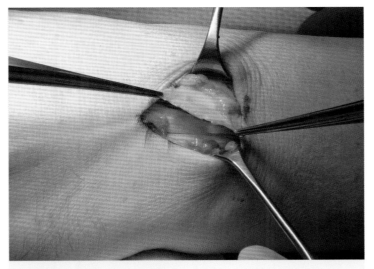

Fig. 2.22 The proximal and distal ends of the extensor retinaculum are identified and it is incised longitudinally parallel to the extensor carpi ulnaris tendon.

► **Postoperative aftercare.** Postoperative radiography. Immobilize the joint in a palmar forearm plaster splint until wound healing is complete. Administer active and passive physical exercise therapy.

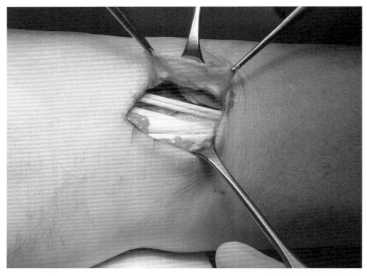

Fig. 2.23 A meticulous tenosynovectomy and joint capsulotomy with extensive articulosynovectomy are performed.

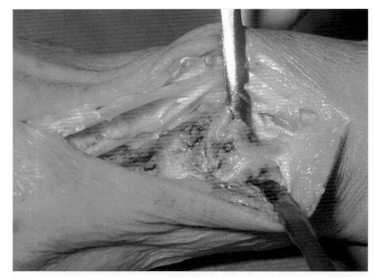

Fig. 2.24 The capsule is opened longitudinally over the ulnar head and an extensive synovectomy is performed. Ulnar head destruction is demonstrated using two Hohmann elevators.

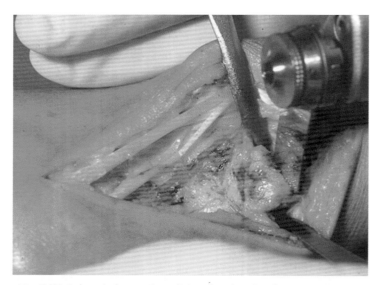

Fig. 2.25 Subcapital resection of the ulnar head is done using an oscillating saw. The synovectomy is then completed in the lower portion of the joint as well.

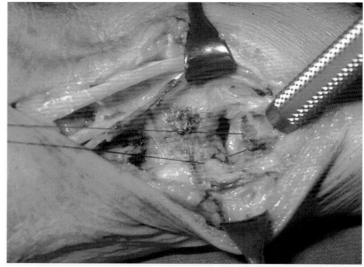

Fig. 2.26 The ulnar stump is repositioned with a tamper and the capsule is reconstructed.

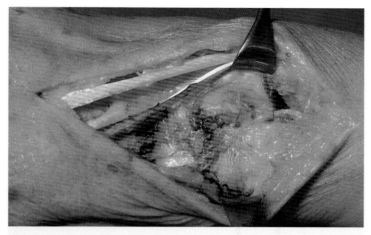

Fig. 2.27 The palmarly subluxed extensor carpi ulnaris muscle tendon is repositioned.

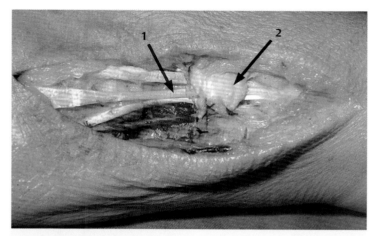

Fig. 2.28 The extensor retinaculum is closed and the incision is sutured in layers. 1, Repositioning the tendons. 2, Extensor retinaculum.

2.2.4 Wrist Prosthesis

▶ **Indication.** Larsen III–V destruction with significant clinical symptoms. Absence of severe axial deformities. No wrist instability (function-sparing procedures such as radiolunate arthrodesis are no longer possible).

▶ **Specific disclosures for patient consent.** Prosthesis loosening or dislocation. Tendon rupture (also secondary). Loss of wrist joint function. Bone fracture/perforation. Damage to sensory nerve branches.

▶ **Instruments.** Prosthesis system from the manufacturer of choice. Standard hand surgery set.

▶ **Position.** Supine. Hand table. The hand should be extended as far as possible onto the hand table. A radiograph may be needed.

▶ **Approach.** See ▶ Fig. 2.29, ▶ Fig. 2.30.

▶ **Wrist prosthesis system (Maestro, Biomet):**
• Carpal plates in eight sizes; capitate stems in three different lengths; carpal heads in three different heights to allow for wrist balancing.
• Scaphoid augments in various sizes.
• Anatomically contoured radial plates in two sizes with four different radial stem sizes.

▶ **Surgical technique.** See ▶ Fig. 2.29, ▶ Fig. 2.30, ▶ Fig. 2.31, ▶ Fig. 2.32, ▶ Fig. 2.33, ▶ Fig. 2.34, ▶ Fig. 2.35, ▶ Fig. 2.36, ▶ Fig. 2.37, ▶ Fig. 2.38, ▶ Fig. 2.39, ▶ Fig. 2.40, ▶ Fig. 2.41, ▶ Fig. 2.42, ▶ Fig. 2.43, ▶ Fig. 2.44, ▶ Fig. 2.45, ▶ Fig. 2.46, ▶ Fig. 2.47.

▶ **Postoperative aftercare.** See ▶ Fig. 2.48, ▶ Fig. 2.49. Immediate full range of motion mobilization (caveat: no shoulder immobilization!). Early finger exercises. Palmar splint for 1 to 3 weeks.

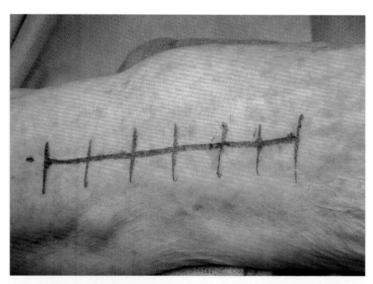

Fig. 2.29 A longitudinal skin incision is made extending from the second or third interdigital space down the ulnar aspect of the wrist joint. A midline incision avoids the radial and ulnar sensory nerve branches.

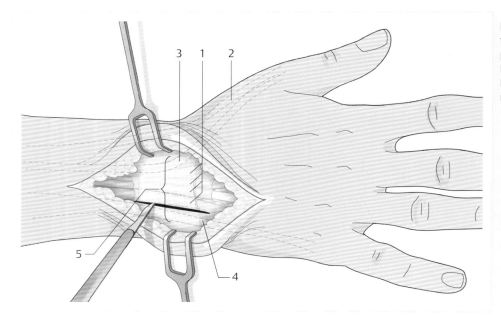

Fig. 2.30 The extensor retinaculum is divided at the level of the fourth extensor tendon compartment. 1, Extensor digitorum muscle. 2, Extensor pollicis brevis muscle. 3, EPL muscle. 4, Extensor digiti minimi muscle. 5, Extensor retinaculum.

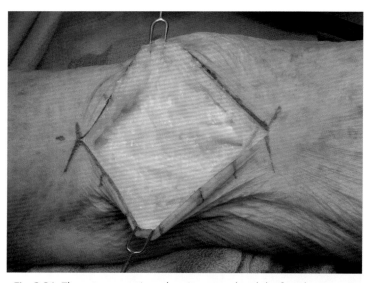

Fig. 2.31 The extensor retinaculum is exposed and the fourth extensor tendon compartment is dissected free. The sensory nerve branches are avoided (exposing the nerves is not essential).

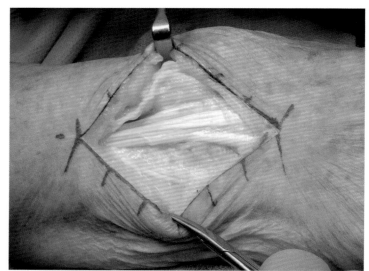

Fig. 2.32 The extensor retinaculum is divided over the fourth extensor tendon compartment so that an ulnar strip remains. This can be used later if needed to reposition the extensor carpi ulnaris in the event of a subluxed tendon.

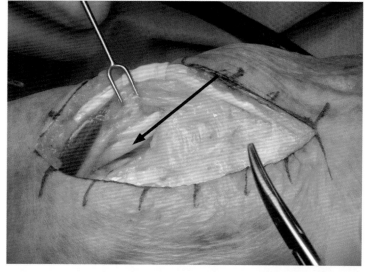

Fig. 2.33 Start of extensor tendon synovectomy. This is accomplished mainly with Luer and Stellbrink rongeurs. The remaining tendon compartments, I–III and V, are exposed. EPL on the dorsal tubercle of radius (Lister's tubercle) (arrow).

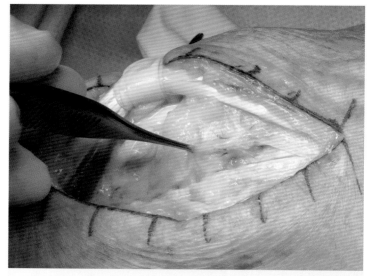

Fig. 2.34 A glove finger and clamp are fastened around the extensor tendons so that they can be held to the side (restraint system). The interosseous nerve of the radial nerve is exposed (forceps). The wrist is denervated by excising ca. 1 cm of the nerve and coagulating the nerve stump.

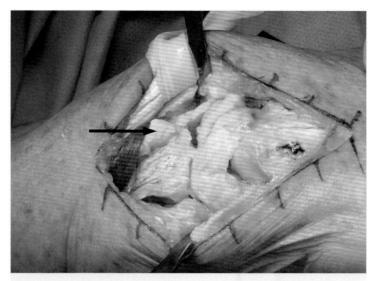

Fig. 2.35 A T-shaped capsulotomy is performed and the capsule is detached from the radius. The capsule is released and the entire damaged wrist joint is revealed. Lister's tubercle (arrow) is shaved flat. It frequently has very sharp edges and can lead to a rupture of the EPL.

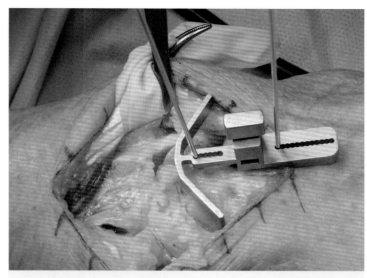

Fig. 2.36 The carpal resection guide is positioned. It is oriented in a direction parallel to the long axis of the third metacarpal. A judicious resection is crucial. The ulnar wing of the guide is aligned with the triquetrum hamate joint and the radial wing bisects the distal third of the scaphoid.

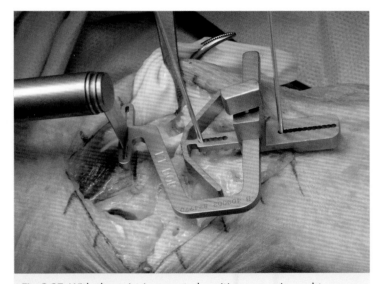

Fig. 2.37 With the wrist in a neutral position, a saw is used to score the radial reference line. This serves as a marker for the resection level of the radius later in the procedure.

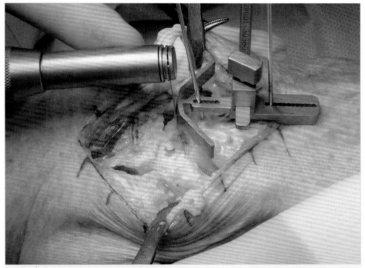

Fig. 2.38 Resection of the scaphoid and capitate head and along the triquetrum edge is accomplished using the carpal resection guide.

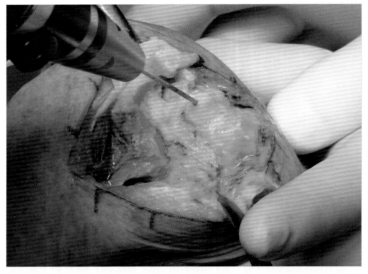

Fig. 2.39 The wrist is opened. The entry point is marked with a K-wire. If there is doubt, a fluoroscopy image is useful.

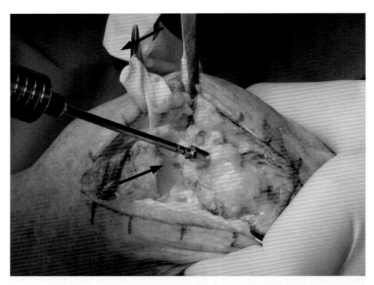

Fig. 2.40 The center opening is bored with a reamer placed over the K-wire. Arrow indicates the radius.

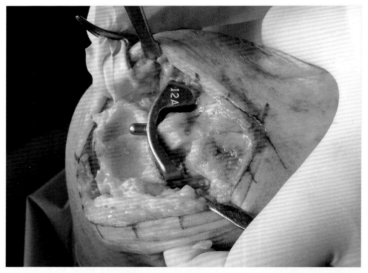

Fig. 2.41 The prosthesis components are trial fitted and the height of the scaphoid augment is determined.

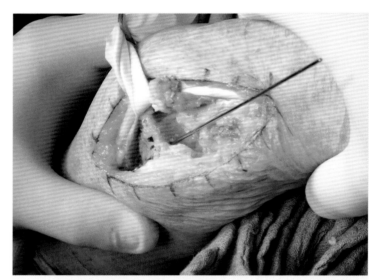

Fig. 2.42 With the wrist in flexion, the radial entry point is created with a K-wire near the center in close proximity to Lister's tubercle. Fluoroscopy helps confirm position. The opening is widened by drilling over the K-wire and then using a radius reamer.

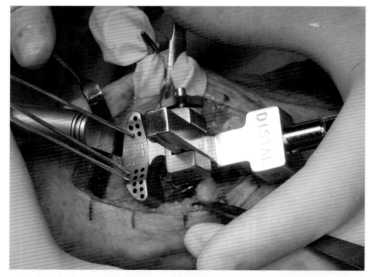

Fig. 2.43 With the reamer kept in place, the resection guide is inserted over the boom.

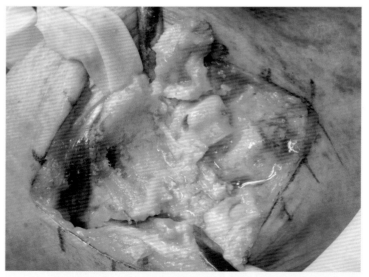

Fig. 2.44 A broach is used as the final step in preparing the radius canal entrance.

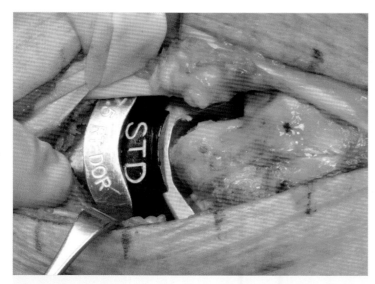

Fig. 2.45 Trial implantation. First the standard size carpal head is inserted. The stability is evaluated and, if necessary, a larger + 2 or + 4 carpal head is inserted. Intraoperative fluoroscopy with an image intensifier is used. If the soft tissues are under too much tension, the radius is further resected.

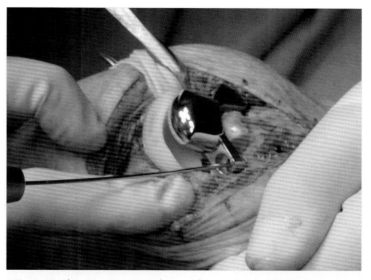

Fig. 2.46 The permanent implant anchoring screw is drilled.

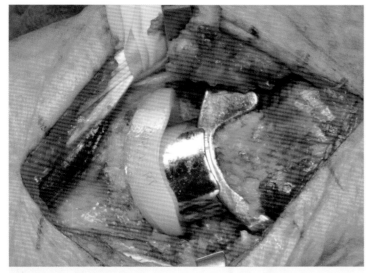

Fig. 2.47 Implanted prosthesis. Cancellous bone is obtained from the resected segments and applied to the eroded bone using compression.

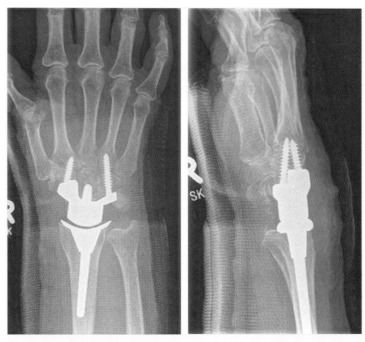

Fig. 2.48 Postoperative radiograph.

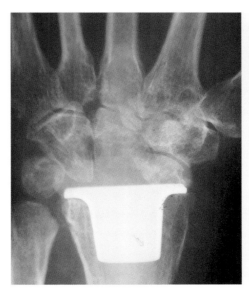

Fig. 2.49 An alternative to joint replacement and a potential possibility for revision surgery: Swanson prosthesis.

2.2.5 Mannerfelt Wrist Arthrodesis

▶ **Indication.** Advanced Larsen IV–V radiocarpal and midcarpal destruction. Simmen type III advanced instability with ulnar drift and palmar subluxation. This is particularly appropriate for fixing the dominant hand in 10 to 20° extension. If needed, the contralateral hand can then be fixed in a neutral position or fitted for a prosthesis.

▶ **Specific disclosures for patient consent.** Postoperative wrist joint function. Delayed or failed bone healing. Hardware dislocation or breakage. Fracture. Damage to sensory nerve branches. Tendon rupture (also secondary).

▶ **Instruments.** Standard hand surgery set; intramedullary hook-end nail (Rush pin). Alternative: plate fixation arthrodesis. Fluoroscopy equipment.

▶ **Position.** Supine. Hand table. The hand should be extended as far as possible onto the hand table. A radiograph may be needed.

▶ **Specifics.** The bones are frequently very osteoporotic.

▶ **Approach.** A dorsal longitudinal incision is made starting over the third metacarpal and extending to the wrist along the ulnar axis.

▶ **Key steps.** Reposition the wrist joint. Completely decorticate the joint surfaces. Prebend the hook-end nail to ca. 50° at the level of the wrist (clinically there will still be 20° of extension left postoperatively). Insert the nail on the ulnar side of the base of the third metacarpal via a bone window.

▶ **Surgical technique.** See ▶ Fig. 2.50, ▶ Fig. 2.51, ▶ Fig. 2.52, ▶ Fig. 2.53, ▶ Fig. 2.54, ▶ Fig. 2.55, ▶ Fig. 2.56, ▶ Fig. 2.57, ▶ Fig. 2.58, ▶ Fig. 2.59, ▶ Fig. 2.60, ▶ Fig. 2.61.

▶ **Postoperative aftercare.** Postoperative radiography. A palmar forearm plaster splint should be applied until wound healing is complete, then circular forearm cast for an additional 4 weeks.

▶ **Alternative.** Plate fixation arthrodesis (▶ Fig. 2.62, ▶ Fig. 2.63).

▶ **Specific disclosures for patient consent.** Extensor tendon problems in the rheumatoid wrist.

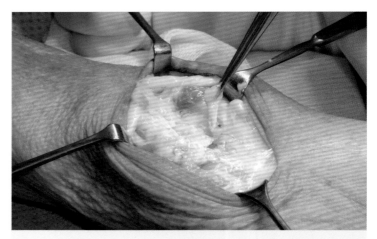

Fig. 2.50 After identifying the distal and proximal ends, the extensor retinaculum is divided longitudinally overlying the fourth extensor tendon compartment, taking care to protect the sensory nerves.

Fig. 2.51 The DRUJ capsule is opened with a longitudinal incision and a synovectomy is performed.

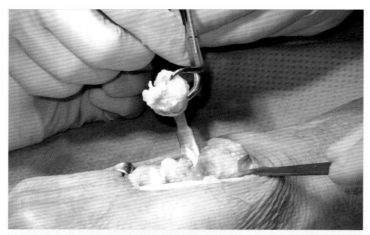

Fig. 2.52 Ulnar head resection.

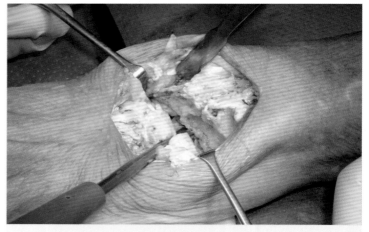

Fig. 2.53 The wrist joint capsule is opened via a flap incision followed by synovectomy and complete decortication of the joint surfaces. Longitudinal traction of the wrist joint and, if needed, palmar flexion facilitate exposure of the joint surfaces. The interosseous (radial) nerve is denervated (see also Chapter 2.2.4).

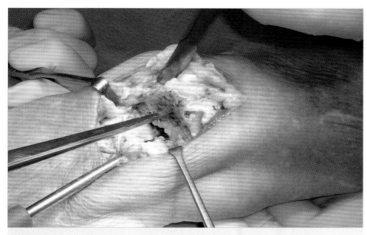

Fig. 2.54 An awl is used to preform the passage before the nail is inserted into the radius.

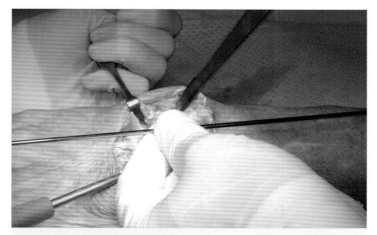

Fig. 2.55 The appropriate length and diameter of the nail are determined.

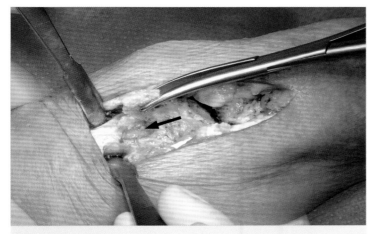

Fig. 2.56 The third metacarpal is exposed (arrow) by placing two Hohmann elevators behind it. A windowlike opening is made in the distal third quarter for insertion of the nail.

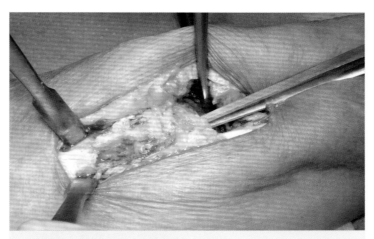

Fig. 2.57 An awl is used to continue preparing the third metacarpal for the Rush pin.

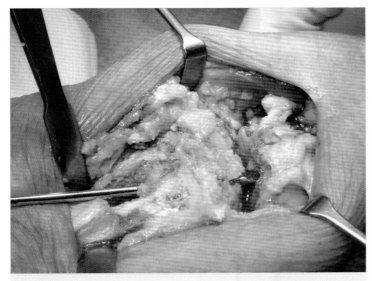

Fig. 2.58 The nail is inserted distally after prebending it to conform to the desired wrist position.

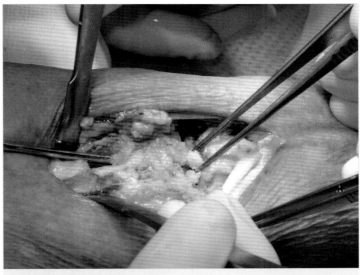

Fig. 2.59 Cancellous bone, obtained from the resected ulnar head, is placed into the wrist joint.

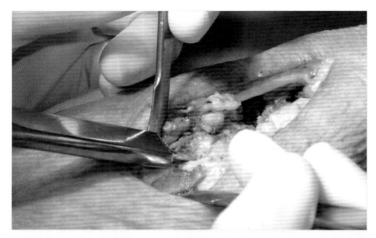

Fig. 2.60 The nail is driven in completely. If necessary, staples can be inserted for additional (rotational) stabilization.

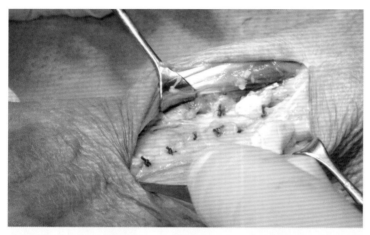

Fig. 2.61 The wrist capsule is sutured and the wound is closed in layers.

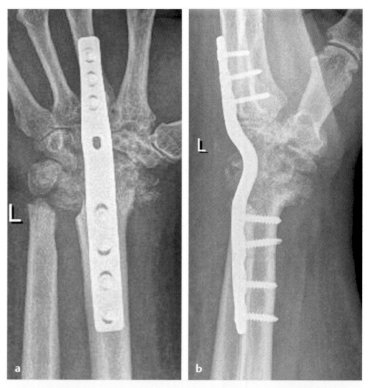

Fig. 2.62 (a,b) Plate fixation arthrodesis with a 2.7-mm distal screw and a 3.5-mm proximal screw.

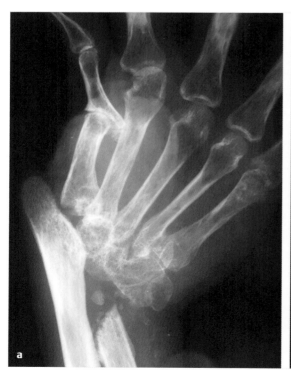
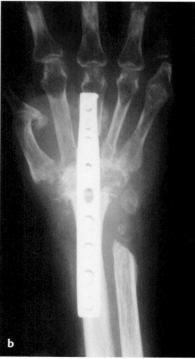

Fig. 2.63 (a,b) Wrist subluxation. There is impending perforation of the skin overlying the ulnar head. An arthrodesis with plate osteosynthesis and simultaneous radial shortening osteotomy was performed, followed by a lateral oblique ulnar osteotomy.

2.3 Tendons

2.3.1 Flexor Tendon Synovitis in the Carpal Tunnel

▶ **Indication.** Tenosynovitis in the flexor tendon canal; possible median nerve entrapment. Persistence of tendon sheath swelling longer than 8 to12 weeks despite adjustment of medical therapy and after appropriate cortisone injection into the carpal tunnel. Additional neurologic examination as indicated.

▶ **Specific disclosures for patient consent.** Median nerve injury. Tendon rupture (also secondary). Damage to sensory nerve branches.

▶ **Instruments.** Standard hand surgery set.

▶ **Position.** Supine. Hand table.

▶ **Specifics.** Identification and loop retraction of the median nerve together with the thenar branch is needed. Careful tenosynovectomy of all tendons within the carpal tunnel must be completed.

▶ **Approach.** A longitudinal curved palmar incision is made over the wrist and extended proximally onto the forearm (▶ Fig. 2.64).

▶ **Key steps.** Dissect layer-by-layer down to the palmar aponeurosis and flexor retinaculum. Incise the retinaculum. Expose the median nerve. Dissect the tendons and excise the synovitis.

▶ **Surgical technique.** See ▶ Fig. 2.65, ▶ Fig. 2.66, ▶ Fig. 2.67, ▶ Fig. 2.68.

▶ **Specific complications.** Nerve injury. Recurrence. Tendon rupture.

▶ **Postoperative aftercare.** Immediate full-range mobilization. Early finger and wrist exercises.

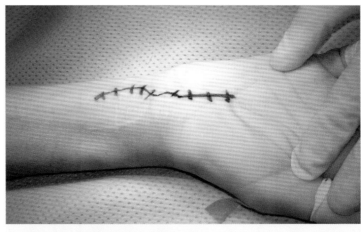

Fig. 2.64 A longitudinal palmar incision is curved proximally over the wrist and continued onto the forearm. The incision is curved in an S-shape over the wrist skin folds. The length of the skin incision depends upon the extent of operative findings.

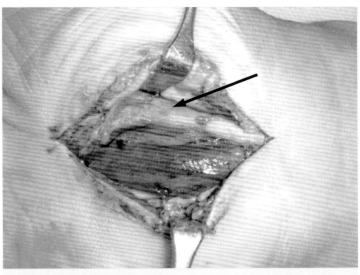

Fig. 2.65 The palmar fascia is exposed distally and divided. The extensor retinaculum is exposed and divided. The median nerve is exposed and retracted (arrow). At the outset, the motor branch of the median nerve is also identified. Severe inflammatory changes of the flexor tendons are apparent.

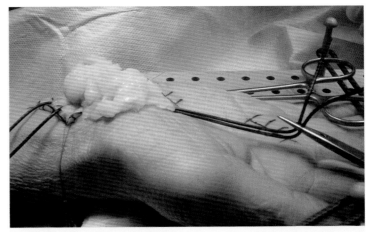

Fig. 2.66 It is crucial, particularly in the presence of pronounced abnormalities, to accurately identify the median nerve and retract it with a loop before performing synovectomy of the flexor tendons.

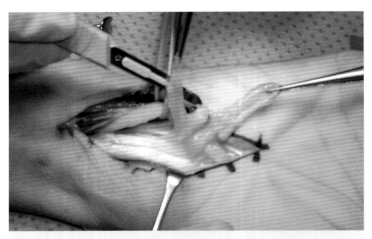

Fig. 2.67 The affected tissue surrounding the tendons is resected. The tendons are individually detached using tendon hooks and can then be easily synovectomized using a Luer. Synovitis that has infiltrated into the tendons is removed with a fresh knife blade. Complete infiltration of the tendons with significantly weakened tendon structure is more difficult to treat. Here it is necessary to weigh performing a complete synovectomy against retaining a relatively stable tendon structure.

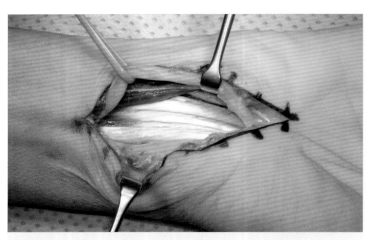

Fig. 2.68 Flexor tendons following complete synovectomy.

2.3.2 Finger and Metacarpal Flexor Tendon Synovectomy

▶ **Indication.** Tenosynovitis of the flexor tendons of the metacarpals and finger canals. Persistence of swelling longer than 8 to 12 weeks despite optimization of medication therapy.

▶ **Specific disclosures for patient consent.** Tendon rupture (also secondary). Injury to motor and sensory nerve branches.

▶ **Instruments.** Standard hand surgery set. Surgical loupes.

▶ **Position.** Supine. Hand table. See also ▶ Fig. 2.70.

▶ **Specifics.** Careful preservation of the A2 and A4 anular ligaments is necessary. Caveat: aberrant (intersecting) finger nerves!

▶ **Approach.** Use a transverse incision if A1 anular synovitis is present or if multiple flexor tendons are involved. A Bruner's zigzag incision is used if there is significant proximal and distal extension of synovitis. See also ▶ Fig. 2.69, ▶ Fig. 2.74.

▶ **Key steps.** For deep dissection: protect the neurovascular structures. Dissect the flexor tendon canal in the midpalmar region of the fingers.

▶ **Surgical technique.** See ▶ Fig. 2.71, ▶ Fig. 2.72, ▶ Fig. 2.73, ▶ Fig. 2.74, ▶ Fig. 2.75, ▶ Fig. 2.76, ▶ Fig. 2.77, ▶ Fig. 2.78, ▶ Fig. 2.79.

▶ **Specific complications.** Nerve injury. Recurrence. Tendon rupture (early/late). Incompetent finger flexor pulley system.

▶ **Postoperative aftercare.** Immediate full-range mobilization. Early finger and wrist exercise.

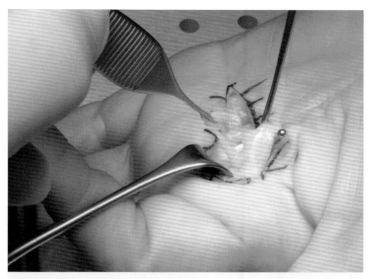

Fig. 2.69 A transverse skin incision is used for isolated findings (which should be verified ultrasonographically).

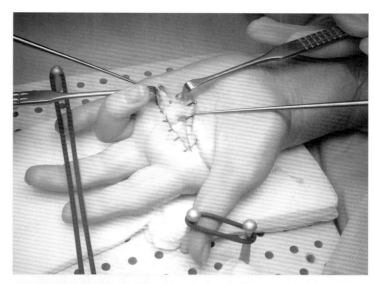

Fig. 2.70 The hand is positioned on the hand table using a "lead hand." If multiple flexor tendons are affected, the transverse skin incision is extended. Depending upon intraoperative findings, the affected fingers are removed from the positioning device to allow better exposure.

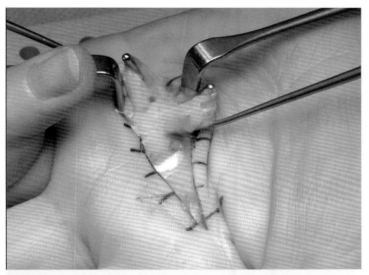

Fig. 2.71 The flexor tendon is exposed via blunt dissection with scissors. The A1 anular ligament is exposed by dissecting in a longitudinal direction along the tendon, taking care to protect the vascular and nerve supply. Synovitis is already bulging proximally and distally out of the flexor tendon canal.

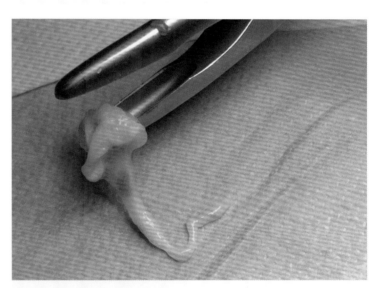

Fig. 2.72 Excised synovitis.

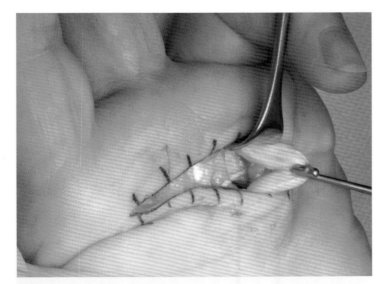

Fig. 2.73 The tendons are lifted using a tendon hook and can then be thoroughly stripped of the inflammatory tissue.

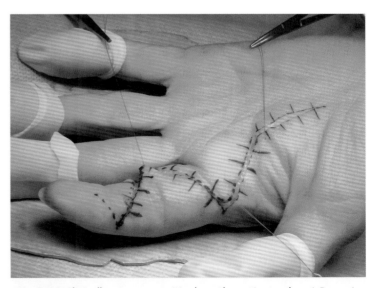

Fig. 2.74 Clinically severe synovitis along the entire tendon. A Bruner's zig-zag shaped incision is made beginning at the PIP joint and extending onto the palm. The incision is marked beforehand.

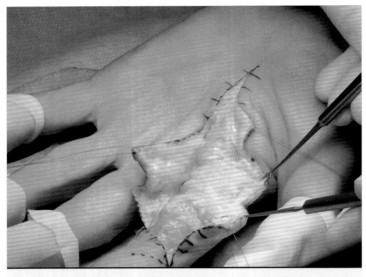

Fig. 2.75 The deep tissue is accessed via layer-by-layer dissection. The skin edges are secured with retaining sutures.

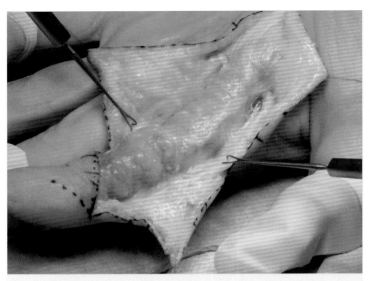

Fig. 2.76 The exposed flexor tendon canal with severely inflamed tendon sheaths.

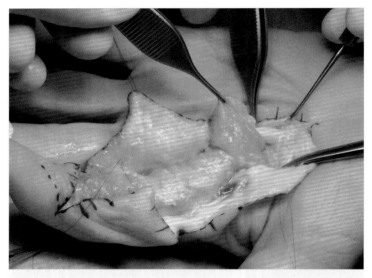

Fig. 2.77 The flexor tendon canal is opened while preserving the easily recognizable neurovascular structures. Illustrated here: pronounced flexor tendon synovitis.

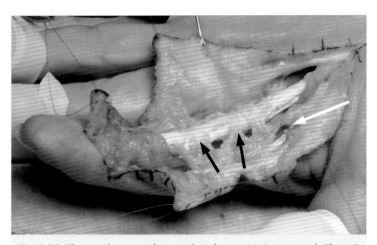

Fig. 2.78 The tendons are dissected and synovitis is resected. The A2 and A4 anular ligaments are preserved (black arrows). The A1 anular ligament is reconstructed if necessary, taking care not to create a stenosis. White arrow indicates the neurovascular bundle.

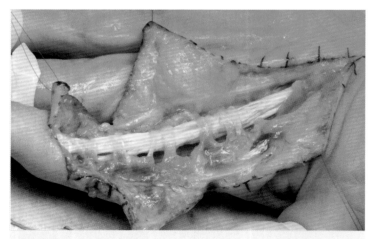

Fig. 2.79 The anular ligaments are exposed. These are severely weakened due to the synovitis.

2.3.3 Wrist Extensor Tendon Synovectomy

▶ **Indication.** Tenosynovitis of the wrist extensor tendons. Persistent swelling longer than 6 to 12 weeks despite optimization of medication therapy and after local treatment (including injection, particularly peritendoneal). This procedure is often performed simultaneously with wrist synovectomy. See also ▶ Fig. 2.80.

▶ **Specific disclosures for patient consent.** Tendon rupture (also secondary). Loss of finger extension.

▶ **Instruments.** Standard hand surgery set.

▶ **Position.** Supine. Hand table.

▶ **Approach.** See ▶ Fig. 2.81.

▶ **Key steps.** The posterior interosseous nerve (radial nerve branch) is resected to reduce wrist joint capsular pain. Excision of Lister's tubercle (distal radial tubercle) may be necessary.

▶ **Surgical technique.** See ▶ Fig. 2.82, ▶ Fig. 2.83, ▶ Fig. 2.84.

▶ **Postoperative aftercare.** Immediate full-range mobilization. Early finger and wrist exercise. Active and passive physical therapy.

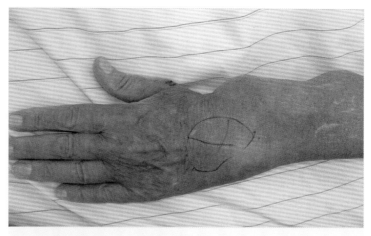

Fig. 2.80 Pronounced dorsal (and radial) tenosynovitis.

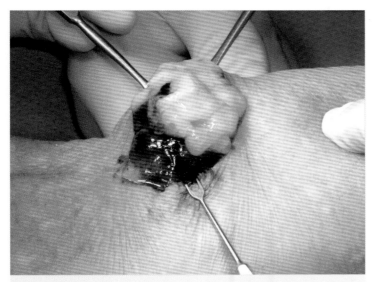

Fig. 2.81 A longitudinal dorsal incision is made over the wrist. Alternatively, an oblique incision can be made from the distal radius to the proximal ulnar region. Smaller incisions are permissible even in cases of extensive involvement.

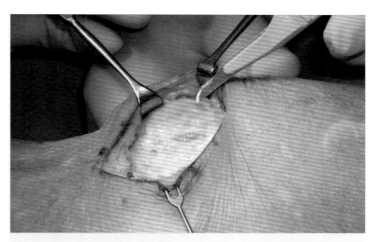

Fig. 2.82 The tissue is dissected in layers down to the extensor retinaculum, which is split longitudinally overlying the fourth extensor tendon compartment.

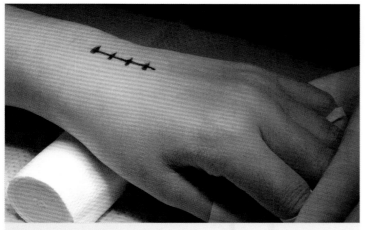

Fig. 2.83 Synovitis surrounding the extensor tendons is exposed and excised. All five extensor tendons are exposed. If Lister's tubercle appears sharp-edged and poses a risk for rupture of the EPL tendon it is resected. The interosseous dorsalis nerve is exposed (see also Chapter 2.2.4), resected 1 cm, and subsequently cauterized. All tendons are inspected and cleaned (lift with a tendon hook). The extensor carpi ulnaris tendon is located and repositioned under the extensor retinaculum in the case of its palmar luxation. (See also Chapter 2.2.3.)

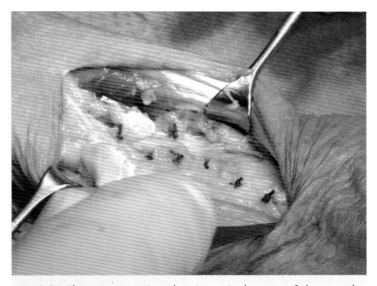

Fig. 2.84 The extensor retinaculum is repaired as part of the wound closure.

2.3.4 Tendon Ruptures

Extensor Tendon Rupture in the Wrist

▶ **Indication.** Rupture of the extensor tendons in the wrist with loss of finger function.

For significant wrist palmar subluxation and supination, a realignment procedure and removal of attached osteophytes may be necessary.

Direct suture of the tendon is usually not possible due to the chronic inflammation and eventual tendon dehiscence. Many patients present late for repair, which also allows tendons to retract.

▶ **Frequent extensor tendon ruptures:**
- EPL. (Reconstruction: indices tendon transfer.)
- Extensor digitorum. (Reconstruction: coupling, indicis transfer, palmaris transplant.)
- Extensor digiti minimi.

▶ **Alternatives.** Arthrodesis of the affected joint.

▶ **Specific disclosures for patient consent.** Loss of finger function. Re-rupture.

▶ **Instruments.** Standard hand surgery set.

▶ **Position.** Supine. Hand table. The hand should be extended as far as possible onto the hand table.

▶ **Approach.** See also radiolunate arthrodesis, Chapter 2.2.2. See ▶ Fig. 2.85.

▶ **Key steps.** Preoperatively verify the presence of the palmaris longus muscle tendon (transplantation may be necessary). Reconstruction is either with a tendon transfer (e.g., indicis proprius), with a side-to-side suture using an intact motor (neighboring) tendon, or with an interposition.

▶ **Surgical technique.** See ▶ Fig. 2.86, ▶ Fig. 2.87, ▶ Fig. 2.88, ▶ Fig. 2.89, ▶ Fig. 2.90, ▶ Fig. 2.91.

▶ **Specific complications.** Re-rupture. Malfunction. Extension deficit.

▶ **Postoperative aftercare.** Immediate full-range mobilization. Early gentle finger exercises. Palmar splint for 1 to 3 weeks, dynamic finger extension splint as needed.

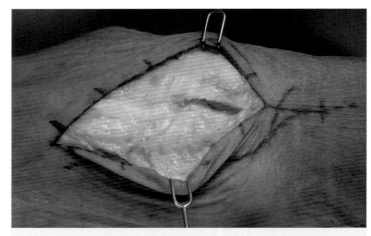

Fig. 2.85 A dorsal longitudinal incision is made over the fourth extensor tendon compartment. Cauliflower-like swelling of the tissue surrounding the rupture.

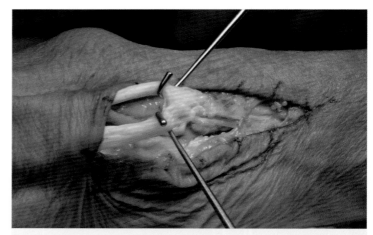

Fig. 2.86 The extensor digitorum distal tendon stumps are identified and exposed.

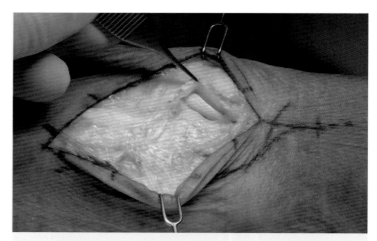

Fig. 2.87 The extensor digitorum proximal tendon stumps are identified.

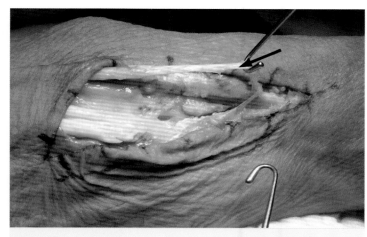

Fig. 2.88 Function of the extensor tendons is evaluated; these clearly appear eroded (arrow) and are also at risk for rupture.

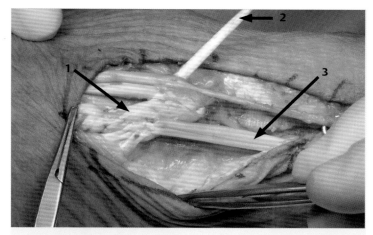

Fig. 2.89 A side-to-side coupling of the ruptured tendon stumps (1) onto the remaining tendons of the extensor digitorum communis muscle is performed. For reinforcement, a free palmaris longus tendon muscle transplant is attached (2). Preserved extensor digitorum tendon (3).

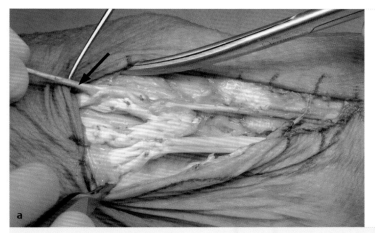

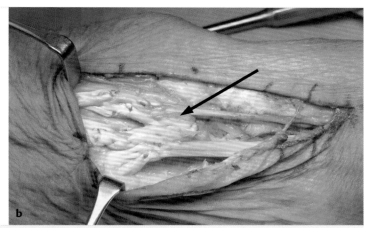

Fig. 2.90 (a,b) The eroded tendons, at risk for rupture, are reinforced with a free transplant from the palmaris longus muscle (arrow).

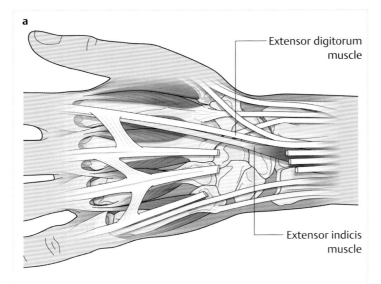

a

Extensor digitorum muscle

Extensor indicis muscle

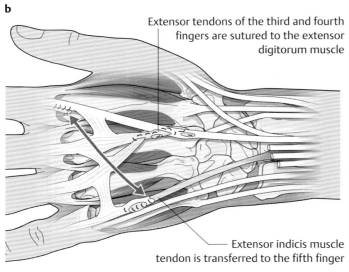

b

Extensor tendons of the third and fourth fingers are sutured to the extensor digitorum muscle

Extensor indicis muscle tendon is transferred to the fifth finger

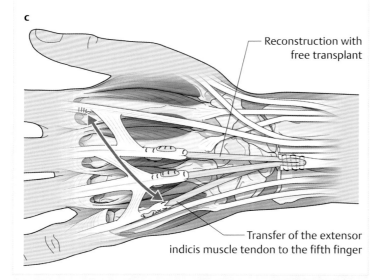

c

Reconstruction with free transplant

Transfer of the extensor indicis muscle tendon to the fifth finger

Fig. 2.91 Schematic for reconstruction of extensor tendon rupture on the third to fifth fingers. **(a)** Preoperative state. **(b)** Status post extensor indicis muscle tendon transfer to the fifth finger and side-to-side suturing of the third and fourth finger extensor tendons to the extensor digitorum muscle tendon. **(c)** Reconstruction using a free transplant.

Flexor Tendon Rupture in the Wrist

▶ **Indication.** Flexor tendon rupture in the wrist region with loss of function in the fingers. Absence of severe alignment deformity or distal articular destruction of the joints. No wrist instability.

A direct tendon suture is usually not feasible due to the long-standing tendon involvement.

For significant wrist palmar subluxation and supination, a realignment procedure and removal of attached osteophytes may be necessary.

▶ **Alternative.** Arthrodesis of the affected joint.

▶ **Specific disclosures for patient consent.** Tendon (re-)rupture (secondary also). Functional deficits in the wrist.

▶ **Instruments.** Standard hand surgery set.

▶ **Position.** Supine. Hand table. See ▶ Fig. 2.92.

▶ **Approach.** Curved palmar incision extending to the carpal tunnel (▶ Fig. 2.93).

▶ **Key steps.** Preoperative verification of the presence of the palmaris longus muscle tendon (transplantation may be necessary). Reconstruction either with tendon interposition over a direct suture or over a side-to-side suture with an intact motor (neighboring) tendon.

▶ **Surgical technique.** See ▶ Fig. 2.93, ▶ Fig. 2.94, ▶ Fig. 2.95.

▶ **Specific complications.** Re-rupture. Incompetence of tendon reconstruction.

▶ **Postoperative aftercare.** Immediate full-range mobilization. Early finger exercises without load. Palmar splint for 1 to 3 weeks; Kleinert splint if needed.

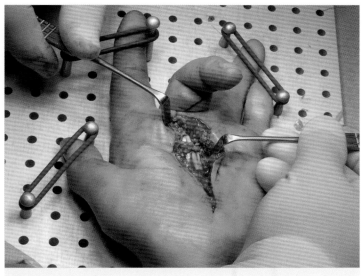

Fig. 2.92 The hand is positioned in a stabilizing device. The flexor tendons are exposed with a Z-shaped approach. Many ruptures located in the wrist region are rarely more distal than the wrist joint.

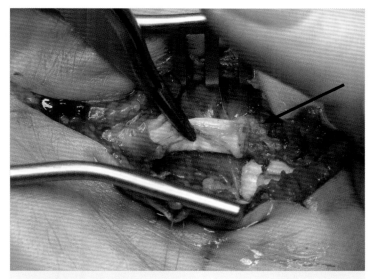

Fig. 2.93 The rupture (longstanding) and its surrounding region are exposed. The tendon stumps (arrow) are debrided.

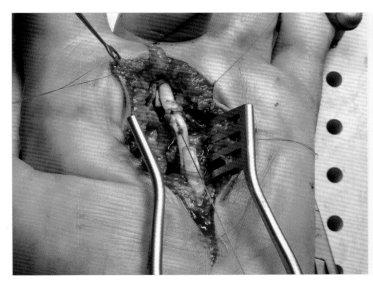

Fig. 2.94 The ruptured tendon is sutured with an interposition from the palmaris longus muscle tendon.

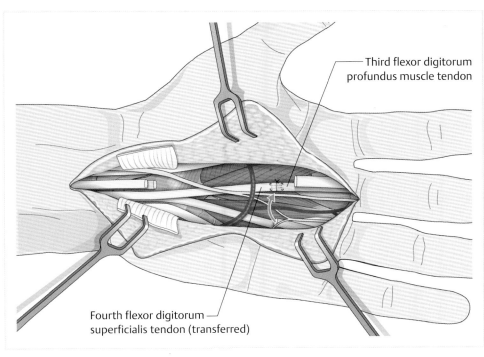

Third flexor digitorum profundus muscle tendon

Fourth flexor digitorum superficialis tendon (transferred)

Fig. 2.95 Schematic of a flexor digitorum superficialis muscle tendon rupture. The necrotic tendon areas and the distal flexor digitorum superficialis muscle are resected. Finally, the fourth flexor digitorum superficialis muscle tendon is transferred onto the third flexor digitorum profundus muscle tendon using a modified Kirchmayr technique with additional epitendinous suture.

2.4 The Finger

2.4.1 Metacarpophalangeal Joint Synovectomy

▶ **Indication.** Metacarpophalangeal (MCP) joint synovitis. Persistent swelling longer than 6 to 12 weeks despite optimization of medication therapy and local treatment (including cortisone infiltration).

As a sole intervention for MCP joint destruction: Larson classification radiological progression no greater than Stage 0–II/III.

▶ **Specific disclosures for patient consent.** Tendon rupture (also secondary); nerve injury.

▶ **Instruments.** Standard hand surgery set.

▶ **Position.** Supine. Hand table.

▶ **Specifics.** Caveat for the skin incision: the extensor hoods lie directly underneath!

If ulnar deviation of the fingers is present, it may be necessary to perform a plication of the radial extensor hood and an open release of the ulnar components.

▶ **Approach.** Dorsal transverse over the MCP joint (▶ Fig. 2.96).

▶ **Key steps.** Use passive longitudinal extension of the surrounding structures intraoperatively to address the palmar joint components.

▶ **Surgical technique.** See ▶ Fig. 2.97

▶ **Specific complications.** Recurrence of articular synovitis. Progressive ulnar deviation of the finger.

▶ **Postoperative aftercare.** Immediate full-range mobilization. Early active and passive finger exercises; ergonomic individually fitted dynamic finger extension splints may be needed with radial traction.

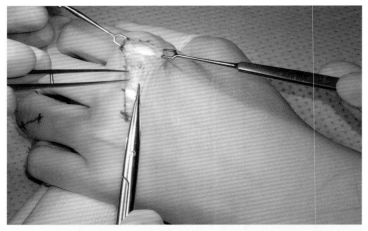

Fig. 2.96 A dorsal transverse incision is made over the MCP joint. The extensor hood is exposed, usually radial to the tendon. In the event of ulnar drift, the extensor tendon is also released on the ulnar side.

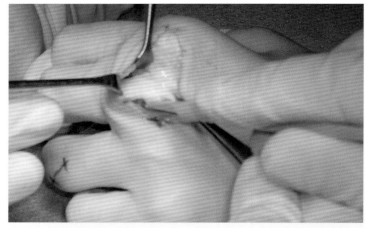

Fig. 2.97 Radial and ulnar incision of extensor hood. For continuation of the procedure see Chapter 2.4.2.

2.4.2 Swanson Prosthesis of Metacarpophalangeal Joint

▶ **Indication.** Larsen III–V MCP joint destruction with significant clinical symptoms. Loss of motion. Ulnar slip of the extensor hood.

No evidence of contractures or axial deformity of the MCP joint that is not passively correctable.

▶ **Specific disclosures for patient consent (here: Swanson prosthesis).** Prosthesis fracture or dislocation. Tendon rupture (also secondary). Loss of finger function. Bone fracture/perforation. Long-term range of motion 0°–20°–70°. Granulomas.

▶ **Instruments.** Prosthesis system from the manufacturer of choice. Standard hand surgery set.

▶ **Position.** Supine. Hand table. A radiograph may be needed.

▶ **Approach.** Dorsal transverse over the MCP joints (▶ Fig. 2.98) (see also Chapter 2.4.1). A longitudinal approach is feasible for a single MCP joint implantation (▶ Fig. 2.99).

▶ **Key steps.** Excise the metacarpal head along a 10° palmar incline. Position the resected surfaces after opening the intramedullary canal. Pay attention to capsular and ligament tension during insertion of the Swanson prosthesis. Reconstruct and re-center the extensor hood with a radial plicating suture and leave the ulnar lamina intertendinea superficialis and the capsule open.

▶ **Specifics.** In the presence of contracture, release the ulnar ligament, detach the radial ligament from its bone insertion, and perform a plicated bone reattachment more radially. Perform a radial transposition of the ulnar interosseous muscles.

▶ **Surgical technique.** See ▶ Fig. 2.100, ▶ Fig. 2.101, ▶ Fig. 2.102, ▶ Fig. 2.103, ▶ Fig. 2.104, ▶ Fig. 2.105, ▶ Fig. 2.106, ▶ Fig. 2.107, ▶ Fig. 2.108, ▶ Fig. 2.109, ▶ Fig. 2.110, ▶ Fig. 2.111.

▶ **Specific complications.** See ▶ Fig. 2.112, ▶ Fig. 2.113. Loss of function. Prosthesis breakage or subluxation. Infection. Recurrence of malposition (particularly ulnar deviation). Instability. Stiffness.

▶ **Postoperative aftercare.** Postoperative radiography. Immediate full-range flexion and extension mobilization. Provide a finger flexion glove. Early finger exercises. Palmar splint for 1 week. Fit with an ergonomic individually customized dynamic finger extension splint with ulnar traction for 3 months.

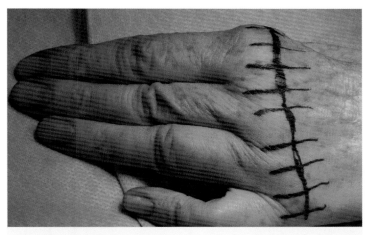

Fig. 2.98 A dorsal transverse approach over the metacarpophalangeal (MCP) joints is used for multiple joint implants.

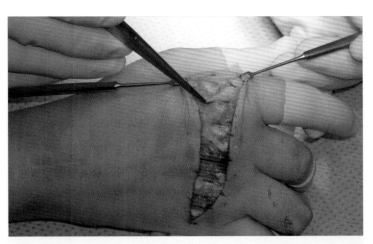

Fig. 2.99 A longitudinal approach is also reasonable for a single MCP joint implant. Here there was no axial deformity, so the extensor aponeurosis was opened longitudinally midline.

Fig. 2.100 The extensor mechanism is exposed and the ulnar side is released. For a luxated extensor mechanism, the radial side is also released for subsequent plication.

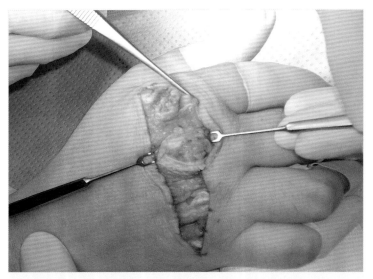

Fig. 2.101 Recentering the joints and balancing the soft tissue is accomplished via a Littler release; see also Chapter 2.4.6.

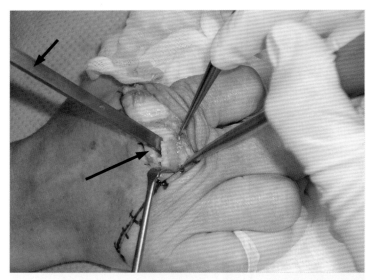

Fig. 2.102 The joint is exposed and arthrotomy along with extensive synovectomy is performed. Osteotomy of the joint surface. Palmar adhesions are removed (rasp in the palmar capsule, arrows).

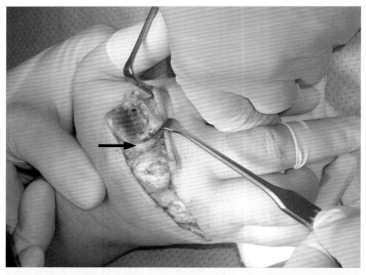

Fig. 2.103 The joint surfaces are sparingly resected using an oscillating saw. The metacarpal head is excised in a slight 10° palmar incline. The collateral ligaments (arrow) are held to the side and protected using a Langenbeck retractor.

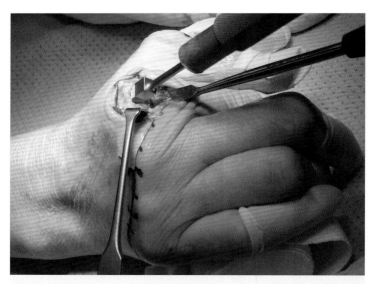

Fig. 2.104 The intramedullary canal is opened and prepared using medullary rasps in progressively larger sizes. The proximal phalanx is prepared in the same manner.

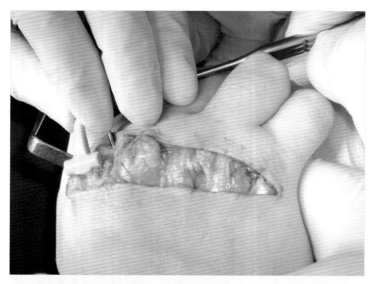

Fig. 2.105 The appropriate prosthesis size is determined: trial implantation.

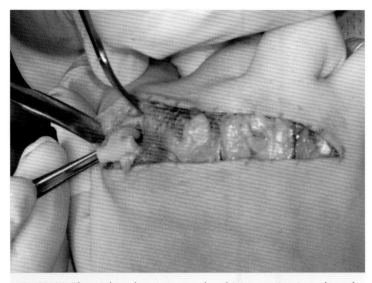

Fig. 2.106 The trial implant is inserted and joint tension is evaluated. The fit and balance of the prosthesis are checked. If needed, the radial collateral ligament is released and transosseous reattachment is carried out before insertion of the implant. For severe deviation, a transposition of the interosseous muscles from ulnar to radial is also an option.

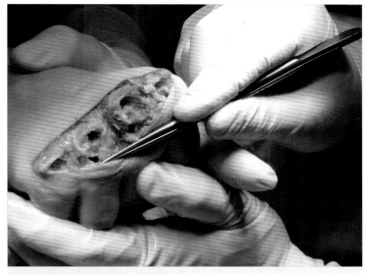

Fig. 2.107 View of the surgical site prepared for prosthesis insertion.

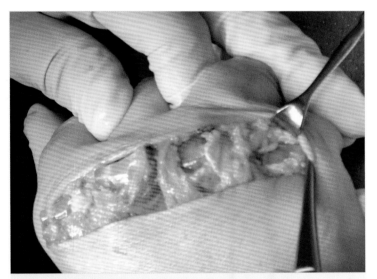

Fig. 2.108 Surgical site with inserted Swanson prosthesis.

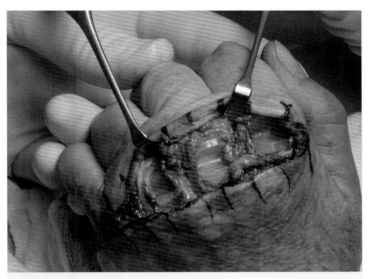

Fig. 2.109 NeuFlex prosthesis as an alternative.

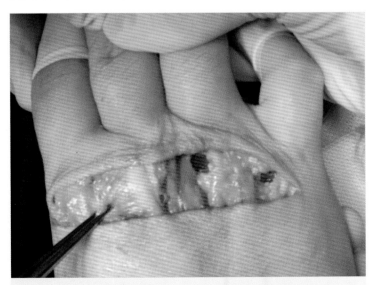

Fig. 2.110 The extensor mechanism is reconstructed and radial plication of the extensor mechanism is carried out (forceps simulate the traction of the plication).

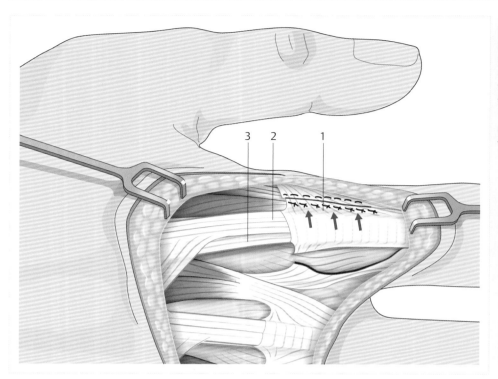

Fig. 2.111 Schematic drawing of a radially plicated suture of the extensor mechanism. For severe contracture, the ulnar interossei muscles are released and transferred to the radial side. At the same time, the radial ligaments are released from the bone and reattached using plication. 1, Lamina intertendinea superficialis radialis (Landsmeer). 2, Extensor digitorum muscle tendon. 3, Extensor indicis muscle tendon.

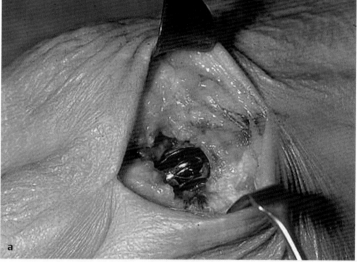
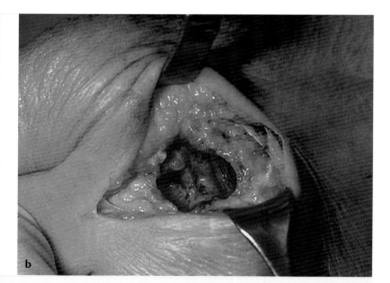

Fig. 2.112 (a,b) Metallosis with a loosened coupled prosthesis.

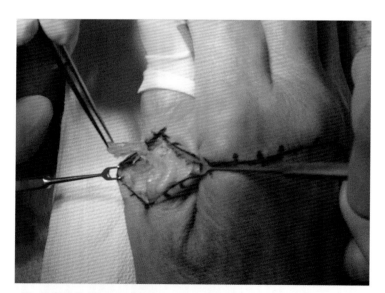

Fig. 2.113 Breakage of a Swanson prosthesis in a thumb.

2.4.3 Proximal Interphalangeal Joint Arthrodesis

▶ **Indication.** Advanced Larsen IV–V destruction with axial deviation or rotational deformity. This is preferred over a prosthesis for destruction of the second PIP joint on the dominant hand (due to the force exerted on it). Fixed swan neck or boutonnière deformity Stage III–IV.

▶ **Specific disclosures for patient consent.** Postoperative joint position (second and third: 20–30° flexion; fourth and fifth: 30–40° flexion); final functional position is determined intraoperatively. Fracture. Component breakage or dislocation. Infection. Shortened finger. Loss of function. Finger-to-palm distance. Pseudarthrosis.

▶ **Instruments.** Standard hand surgery set. 1.0-mm K-wire and 0.8-mm cerclage wire. Cannulated screw. Fluoroscopy equipment.

▶ **Position.** Supine. Hand table. A radiograph may be needed.

▶ **Approach.** Dorsal over the PIP joint (▶ Fig. 2.114, ▶ Fig. 2.115).

▶ **Key steps.** Relocate the joint surfaces according to the desired flexion. For joint position during drilling and insertion of the screw, pay attention to the rotation.

▶ **Surgical technique.** See ▶ Fig. 2.116, ▶ Fig. 2.117, ▶ Fig. 2.118, ▶ Fig. 2.119.

▶ **Alternative.** Tension band osteosynthesis. Identical procedure as for the thumb MCP joint; see Chapter 2.4.5.

▶ **Postoperative aftercare.** Postoperative radiography. Plastic splint for 6 weeks.

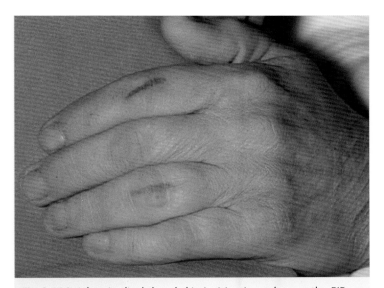

Fig. 2.114 A longitudinal dorsal skin incision is made over the PIP joint. Alternatively, a curved dorsal approach can be used.

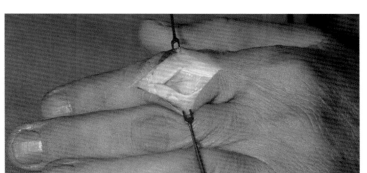

Fig. 2.115 The tractus intermedius is incised longitudinally in the midline.

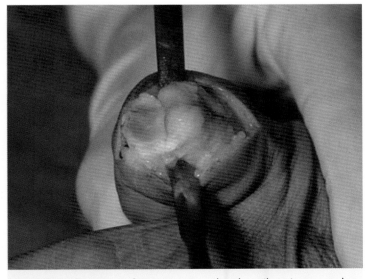

Fig. 2.116 The joint surfaces are exposed and cartilage is removed.

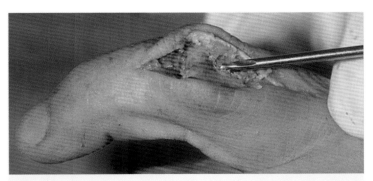

Fig. 2.117 The desired flexion position is set and the screw pilot hole is predrilled.

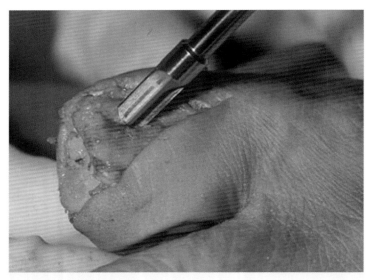

Fig. 2.118 Countersink.

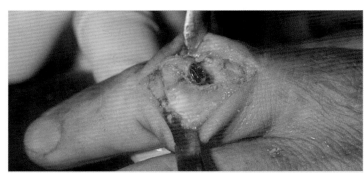

Fig. 2.119 The screw is inserted for joint fixation.

2.4.4 Proximal Interphalangeal Joint Prosthesis

▶ **Indication.** Larsen IV–V destruction with significant clinical symptoms of the third to fifth fingers. Axial deviation. Joint instability.

▶ **Specific disclosures for patient consent.** Prosthesis breakage. Tendon rupture (also secondary). Loss of PIP joint function. Bone fracture/perforation. Granulomas. Instability. Stiffness.

▶ **Instruments.** Prosthesis system from the manufacturer of choice. Standard hand surgery set.

▶ **Position.** Supine. Hand table. A radiograph may be needed.

▶ **Specifics.** Arthrodesis is preferred for the second finger PIP joint on the dominant hand due to the exertional forces!

▶ **Approach.** ▶ Fig. 2.120, see also Chapter 2.4.3. Alternative: palmar or lateral approach.

▶ **Key steps.** Transtendoneal approach to the joint (see also Chapter 2.4.3), or via distal removal of the tractus centralis on the dorsal base of the middle phalanx (then reattached with bone suture), or by cutting the tractus centralis tendon. Position the resected surfaces after opening the medullary canal. Assess capsule and ligament tension during prosthesis insertion.

▶ **Surgical technique.** See ▶ Fig. 2.121, ▶ Fig. 2.122, ▶ Fig. 2.123, ▶ Fig. 2.124, ▶ Fig. 2.125, ▶ Fig. 2.126.

▶ **Alternatives.** Swanson prosthesis.

▶ **Specific complications.** Loss of function. Prosthesis breakage or subluxation. Infection. Malposition. Instability. Stiffness. Granulomas.

▶ **Postoperative aftercare.** Postoperative radiography. Immediate gentle mobilization, specifically the metacarpophalangeal (MCP) and distal interphalangeal (DIP) joints. This is continued over several weeks depending upon the tractus centralis reconstruction and the initial flexion restriction.

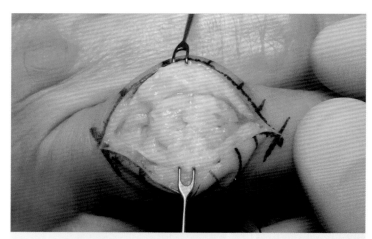

Fig. 2.120 A longitudinal midline incision of the tractus centralis is performed (see also approach for arthrodesis, Chapter 2.4.3).

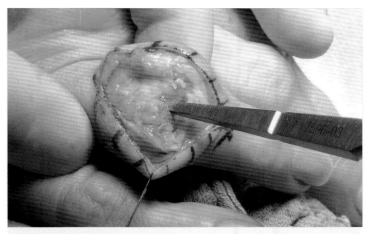

Fig. 2.121 After exposure and removal of cartilage of the proximal joint surfaces, the proximal medullary canal is opened with an awl.

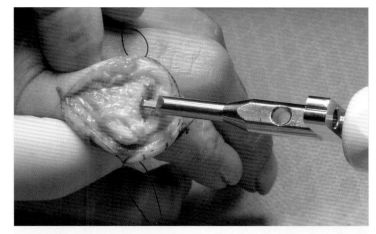

Fig. 2.122 The medullary canal is prepared by inserting rasps of increasing sizes.

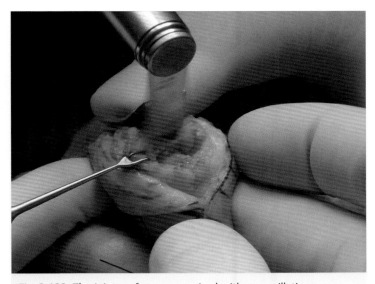

Fig. 2.123 The joint surfaces are excised with an oscillating saw.

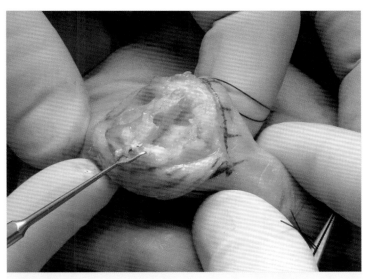

Fig. 2.124 The resected surfaces are aligned with each other.

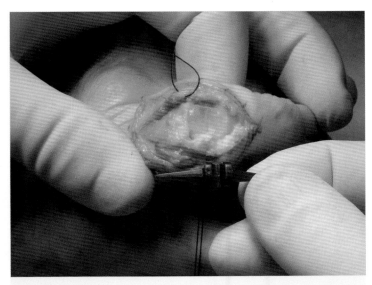

Fig. 2.125 Size is determined using trial implants and the prosthesis is inserted.

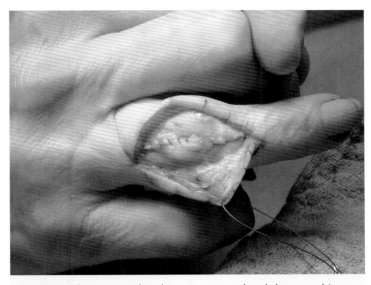

Fig. 2.126 The extensor hood is reconstructed and the wound is closed in layers.

2.4.5 Arthrodesis of the Thumb Metacarpophalangeal Joint

▶ **Indication.** Larsen IV–V destruction. Fixed boutonnière deformity. Disabling instability that reduces function.

▶ **Specific disclosures for patient consent.** Postoperative joint position (10° flexion, mild opposition). Delayed or failed bone healing. Fracture. Component breakage or dislocation. Shortened thumb.

▶ **Instruments.** Standard hand surgery set. 0.8-mm cerclage wire. 1.0-mm K-wire. Fluoroscopy equipment.

▶ **Position.** Supine. Hand table. A radiograph may be needed.

▶ **Approach.** Dorsal. Curved radial incision over the first MCP joint (▶ Fig. 2.127).

▶ **Key steps.** Positioning the thumb: take care to avoid creating an ulnar deviation of the proximal phalanx over the first metacarpal (it is important that the hand can open enough to pick up objects between the thumb and the hand). Mild thumb opposition: thumb pinch tested intraoperatively.

▶ **Surgical technique.** See ▶ Fig. 2.128, ▶ Fig. 2.129, ▶ Fig. 2.130, ▶ Fig. 2.131.

▶ **Alternatives.** Screw fixation arthrodesis; however, this is less stable in osteoporotic bones.

▶ **Postoperative aftercare.** Postoperative radiography. Plastic splint for 6 weeks. The IP joint can be actively and passively mobilized.

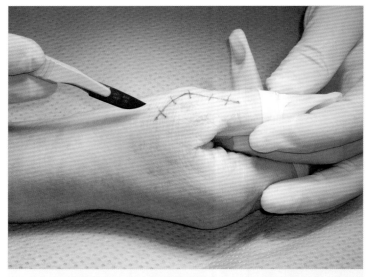

Fig. 2.127 A dorsal curved radial incision is made over the first metacarpophalangeal (MCP) joint.

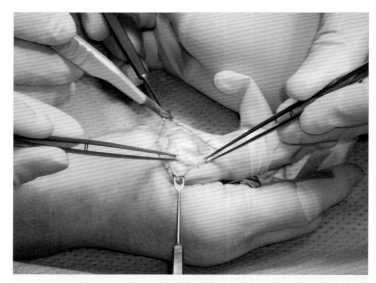

Fig. 2.128 The extensor tendon is held to the side and a longitudinal dorsal capsulotomy is performed.

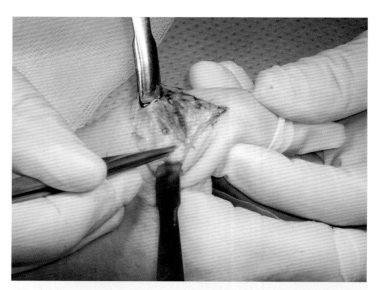

Fig. 2.129 The ligaments are detached so that the proximal phalanx is flexed and the palmar adhesions can be released. The cartilage is removed from the joint surfaces and sparing subchondral débridement is performed.

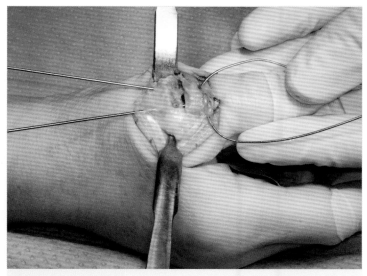

Fig. 2.130 The cerclage wire is introduced into the proximal phalanx base. A short cannula is clamped into the drill and driven transversely through the proximal phalanx. The cerclage wire is inserted and pulled through again using the drill with attached cannula. The osteotomy surfaces are stacked in the desired position (10° flexion). An additional osteotomy inclined radially might be needed in order to open the first commissure, since rheumatic deformity frequently leads to adduction contracture of the thumb. Two thin K-wires, inserted from dorsal proximal to palmar distal, are used to fix this position. Their holes are predrilled to a depth where resistance is met from the opposite cortical layer. Intraoperative fluoroscopy with image intensification is used for confirmation.

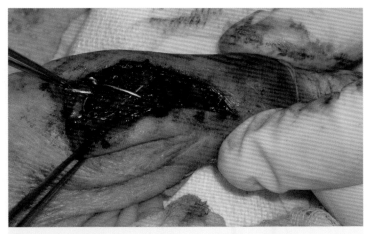

Fig. 2.131 A cerclage wire is wound around the K-wire in a figure-of-eight and twisted into a cerclage closure. The K-wire is bent and shortened. The wound is closed in layers.

2.4.6 Littler's Intrinsic Release of Swan Neck Deformity

The swan neck deformity is much more functionally debilitating than the boutonnière deformity. An imbalance between the flexors and extensors leads to a hyperextended PIP joint and DIP joint flexion. Palmar subluxation of the proximal phalanx causes a shift in the direction of movement of the interosseous and lumbrical muscles.

▶ **Indication.** Loss of finger flexion function in Stage II (active flexion of the PIP joint is no longer possible but can still be achieved passively), see ▶ Fig. 2.132.

▶ **Swan neck deformity classification:**
• Stage I: full active fist closure; consider dermadesis, tenodesis.
• Stage II: Active PIP joint flexion is restricted in certain positions. Passive PIP joint flexion is still possible. PIP joint flexion is influenced by the position of the MCP joint; consider Littler's release, repositioning.
• Stage III: PIP movement is restricted in any position; carry out a flexor digitorum sublimis tendon tenodesis and central slip tenotomy.
• Stage IV: Destruction of joint surfaces. Perform an arthrodesis if not passively correctable.

▶ **Specific disclosures for patient consent.** Stiffness. Recurrence. Progression.

▶ **Instruments.** Standard hand surgery set.

▶ **Position.** Supine. Hand table. Surgical loupes if necessary.

▶ **Specifics.** The swan neck deformity arises from palmar subluxation of the metacarpal phalangeal joints over their respective metacarpals.

▶ **Approach.** Transverse incision over the affected finger's metacarpal. See ▶ Fig. 2.133.

▶ **Key steps.** Subcutaneous exposure of the extensor hood up to the PIP joint via the MCP incision.

▶ **Surgical technique.** See ▶ Fig. 2.134, ▶ Fig. 2.135, ▶ Fig. 2.136, ▶ Fig. 2.137, ▶ Fig. 2.138.

▶ **Specific complications.** Extensor hood injury during incision. Insufficient release of the tractus lateralis (subcutaneously up to the PIP joint in the radial and ulnar tendon spaces) with persistence of the proximal phalanx base palmar subluxation.

▶ **Postoperative aftercare.** Palmar plaster splint up to the mid proximal phalanx for 2 weeks (so that during active flexion the base of the proximal phalanx in the MCP joint is engaged). Following skin suture removal, 3 months in an ergonomic individually fitted dorsal dynamic finger extension splint in which the MCP joint is centered during flexion (radial pull).

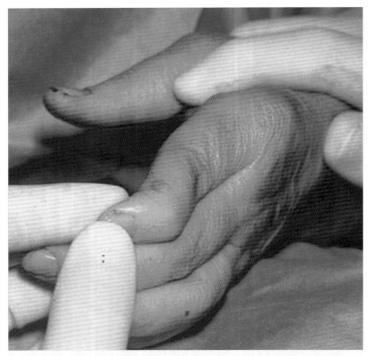

Fig. 2.132 Typical swan neck deformity. The deformity is no longer correctable actively but it is still possible passively.

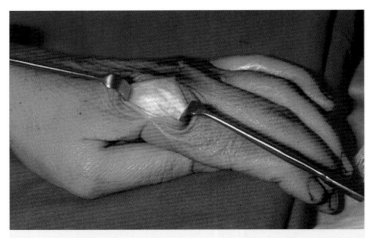

Fig. 2.133 A transverse incision is made over the MCP joint and the extensor tendon is exposed.

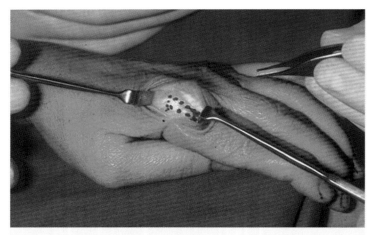

Fig. 2.134 The lamina intertendinealis superficialis is outlined.

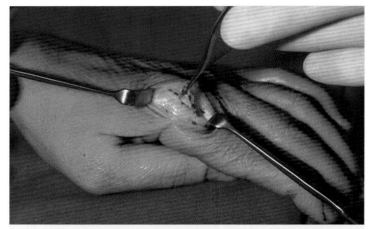

Fig. 2.136 The tendon strip is extracted from the radial and ulnar tendon spaces.

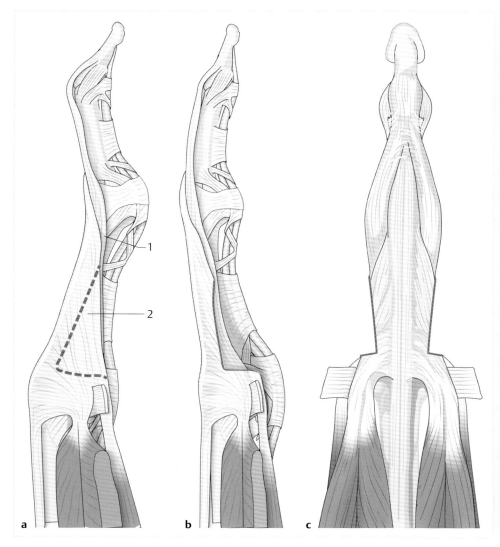

Fig. 2.135 Intrinsic release. **(a)** Radial and ulnar excision of a three-sided tendon window in the lamina intertendineus superficialis (Landsmeer). 1, Oblique retinacular ligament (Landsmeer ligament). 2, Tractus lateralis. **(b)** Status post intrinsic release, from the ulnar view. **(c)** Status post intrinsic release, from the dorsal view.

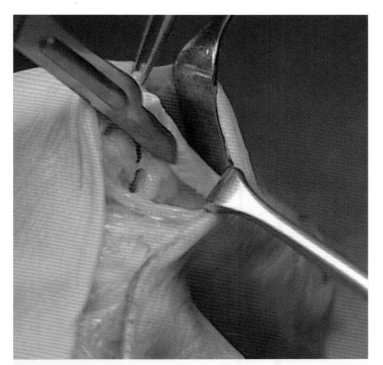

Fig. 2.137 Subcutaneous release of the intrinsic muscles is performed in the space between the tractus centralis and along both sides of the tractus lateralis up to the PIP joint.

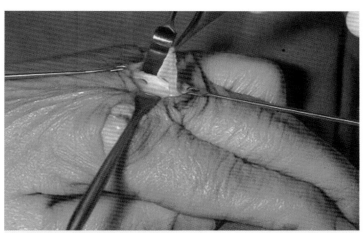

Fig. 2.138 The incised tractus lateralis is exposed.

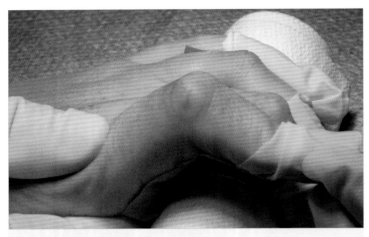

Fig. 2.139 Stage II boutonnière deformity.

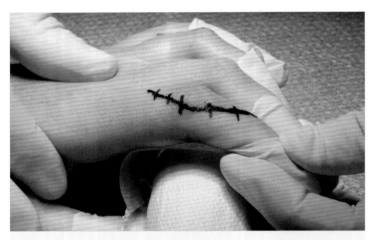

Fig. 2.140 A dorsal longitudinal curved incision is made over the PIP joint.

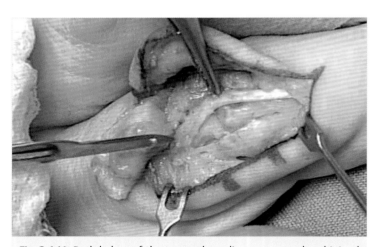

Fig. 2.141 Both halves of the tractus lateralis are prepared and joined dorsally over the PIP joint to close the buttonhole.

2.4.7 Boutonnière Deformity

Boutonnière deformity occurs in up to 30 to 40% of patients. The flexion deformity of the PIP joint with hyperextension of the DIP joint results from extensor apparatus elongation that leads to erosion and displacement.

▶ **Indication.** Synovitis of the PIP joint in Stage II (passive correction still possible), see ▶ Fig. 2.139.

▶ **Classification of boutonnière deformity:**
- Stage I: early flexion deformity, 10 to 15° in the PIP joint. Passively easily correctable—early articulosynovectomy (ASE), central extensor slip plication.
- Stage II: moderate deformity, less than 60° flexion in the PIP joint. Passively easily correctable—ASE, central slip reconstruction.
- Stage III: moderate deformity, less than 60° flexion in PIP joint. Passively no longer completely correctable—stretching with dynamic splinting, subsequent treatment as in Stage II.
- Stage IV: severe fixed flexion deformity—arthrodesis with a fixated flexion position.

▶ **Specific disclosures for patient consent.** Recurrence. Persistence of deformity with impairment of the PIP joint function.

▶ **Instruments.** Standard hand surgery set.

▶ **Position.** Supine. Hand table.

▶ **Approach.** Dorsal longitudinal curved over the PIP joint. See ▶ Fig. 2.140.

▶ **Key steps.** Meticulous preparation of both sides of one half of the tractus lateralis. Synovectomy prior to combining the tractus halves over the PIP joint (closure of the buttonhole). Temporary K-wire stabilization of the PIP joint for 2 to 3 weeks in a corrected position if necessary.

▶ **Surgical technique.** See ▶ Fig. 2.141, ▶ Fig. 2.142, ▶ Fig. 2.143.

▶ **Specific complications.** Failure of the repair with persistent deformity.

▶ **Postoperative aftercare.** Gentle active and passive mobilization of the PIP joint for 6 weeks, so that the tendinoplasty does not elongate.

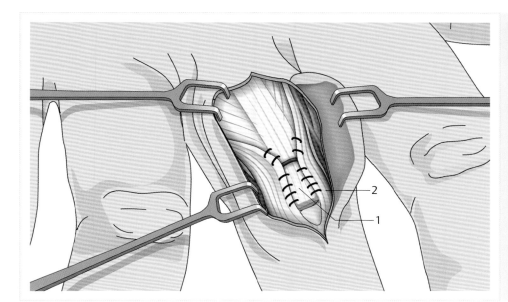

Fig. 2.142 The tractus lateralis is mobilized and repositioned. It is recentered dorsally. 1, Tractus intermedius. 2, Tractus lateralis.

2

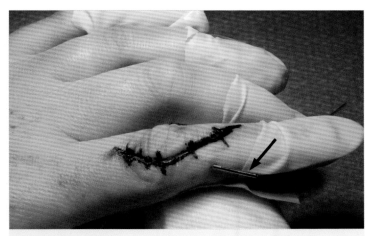

Fig. 2.143 Postoperative spontaneous PIP joint position following closure of the boutonnière deformity. Fixation is performed with a K-wire (arrow).

2.4.8 Trapezium Resection with Suspension Arthroplasty (Destruction of Thumb Carpometacarpal Joint)

▶ **Indication.** Larsen Stage IV–V rhizarthrosis and significant clinical symptoms. First carpometacarpal joint instability with subluxation.

▶ **Specific disclosures for patient consent.** Persistent weakness. Bone fracture. Injury to radial nerve cutaneous sensory branches. Vessel injury (radial artery in the snuffbox).

▶ **Instruments.** Standard hand surgery set. Surgical loupes if necessary.

▶ **Position.** Supine. Hand table. Arrange for radiography.

▶ **Specifics.** Extensor carpi radialis longus (ECRL), flexor carpi radialis longus (FCRL), or abductor pollicis longus (APL) suspension arthroplasty. This intervention cannot correct the MCP joint instability that occurs in conjunction with the thumb saddle joint destruction.

▶ **Approach.** Dorsal oblique or longitudinal incision from the base of MC1 to the base of MC2 as well as a 2-cm-long transverse incision ca. 6 cm proximal to Lister's tubercle (to harvest a one-third portion of the ECRL tendon).

Alternatives: if significant wrist flexion exists, remove the FCRL from the joint (only one skin incision necessary) or the APL using the same incision.

▶ **Key steps.** In the snuff box: loop retraction and protection of the radial artery. H-shaped capsulotomy of the first trapeziometacarpal joint. Complete excision of the trapezium. Two holes are created in the base of MC1 with a 3.5-mm drill to accommodate the tendon graft (note: leave a large enough bone bridge). Expose the MC2 extensor carpi radialis longus muscle insertion site and pass a surgical clamp under the tendon. Then locate the ECRL tendon through a counter-incision proximal to Lister's tubercle. Isolate and split one-third of the tendon and pull through distally with a Halsted clamp to its final insertion site at the base of the second metacarpal. Pass the tendon under the neurovascular structures of the first commissure. Thread through the drill hole. Place the first metacarpal base next to the second metacarpal base, making sure to maintain the thumb length. The first metacarpal base now sits directly next to the second metacarpal base. The harvested tendon is sutured to itself while firmly maintaining this position. Approximately 6 cm of the excess tendon is rolled up into a ball and inserted into the space created from the excised trapezium. A K-wire is placed into the first and second metacarpals temporarily in order to hold the first commissure open and maintain the solid bone structure. The procedure can also be performed without the K-wire.

▶ **Surgical technique.** See ▶ Fig. 2.144, ▶ Fig. 2.145, ▶ Fig. 2.146, ▶ Fig. 2.147, ▶ Fig. 2.148, ▶ Fig. 2.149, ▶ Fig. 2.150, ▶ Fig. 2.151, ▶ Fig. 2.152, ▶ Fig. 2.153, ▶ Fig. 2.154.

▶ **Specific complications.** Radial artery injury. Tendon rupture. Fracture of the bone bridge that the tendon passes through at the first metacarpal base. Loss of thumb length with protrusion of the first metacarpal base into the trapezoid space.

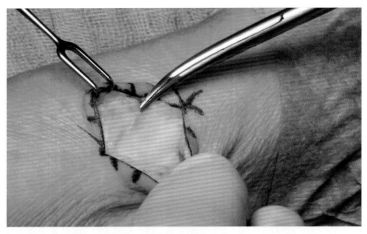

Fig. 2.144 The layers between the abductor pollicis longus and extensor pollicis brevis muscles are dissected down to the trapezio-metacarpal joint.

▶ **Postoperative aftercare.** Postoperative radiography. Immobilize in a cast for 6 weeks; then remove the temporary fixation K-wire. Next begin gentle range of motion exercise with stepwise increases.

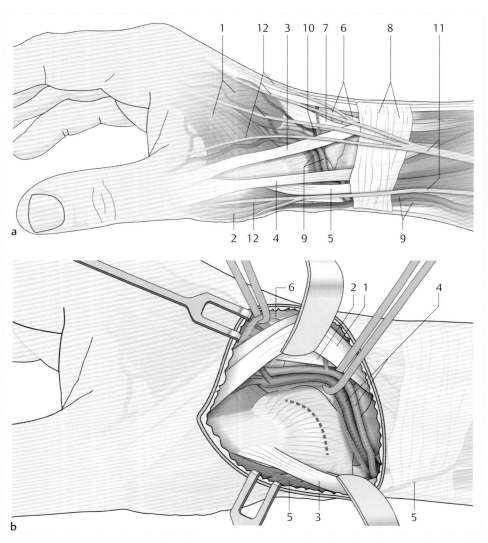

Fig. 2.145 (a) Anatomy of the radial side of the wrist joint. 1, First dorsal interosseous muscle. 2, Abductor pollicis brevis muscle. 3, EPL muscle. 4, Extensor pollicis brevis muscle. 5, Abductor pollicis longus muscle. 6, Extensor carpi radialis brevis muscle. 7, Extensor carpi radialis longus muscle. 8, Extensor retinaculum. 9, Radial artery and vein. 10, Dorsal carpal branch (radial artery). 11, Superficial branch of the radial nerve. 12, Digitalis dorsalis proprius nerve. **(b)** Following exposure and retraction of the radial artery, the joint capsule is opened over the thumb saddle joint along the dotted line. 1, Extensor pollicis brevis muscle. 2, Extensor carpi radialis longus muscle. 3, Abductor pollicis longus muscle. 4, Radial artery and vein. 5, Cephalica pollicis vein. 6, Superficial branch of the radial nerve.

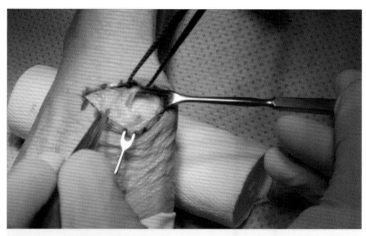

Fig. 2.146 A transverse approach is better for the extensor carpi radialis longus (ECRL). The ECRL is obtained via a second incision. Dissection is performed in layers down to the trapeziometacarpal joint. If needed, the radial artery is exposed proximally and retracted with a loop.

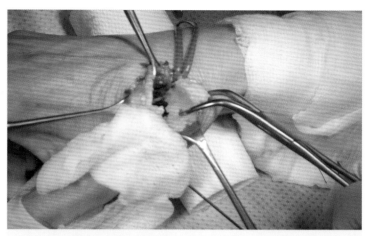

Fig. 2.147 A sharp release of the contracted trapezoid capsular ligament is done under direct visualization. The trapezium is completely excised quite easily using a corkscrew. If significant contracture exists, the trapezium must be osteotomized so that it can be removed.

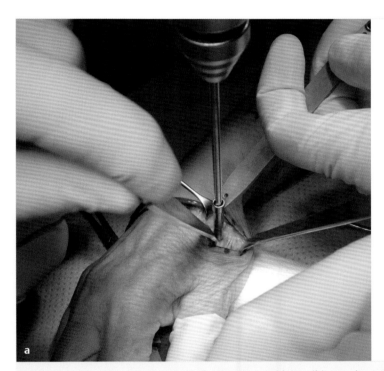

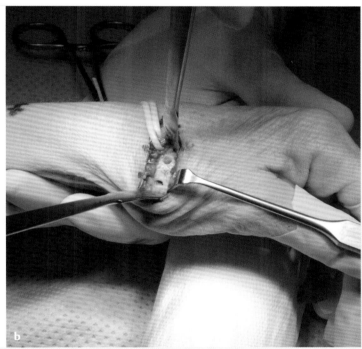

Fig. 2.148 **(a)** Holes drilled into the first metacarpal base. **(b)** An adequately sized bridge must be left between the drilled holes.

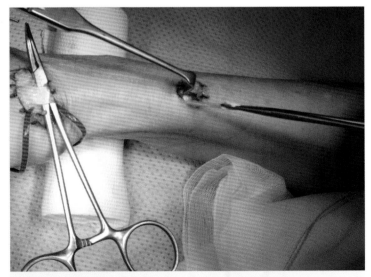

Fig. 2.149 The ECRL tendon is located via the proximal counter-incision. Alternative: APL/FCRL (abductor pollicis longus/flexor carpi radialis longus) suspension arthroplasty.

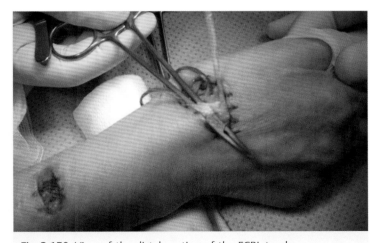

Fig. 2.150 View of the distal portion of the ECRL tendon.

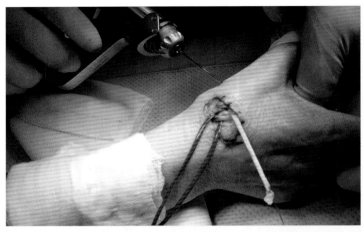

Fig. 2.151 Temporary K-wire fixation of MC1 and MC2 is performed to protect the tendinoplasty.

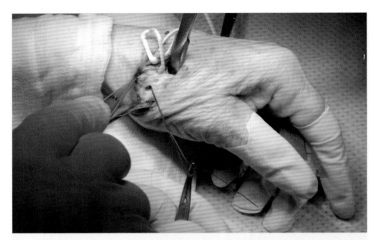

Fig. 2.152 One-third of the ECRL tendon is split off and pulled through distally using a Halsted clamp.

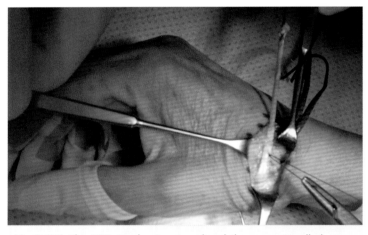

Fig. 2.153 The ECRL tendon is sutured and the excess is rolled up.

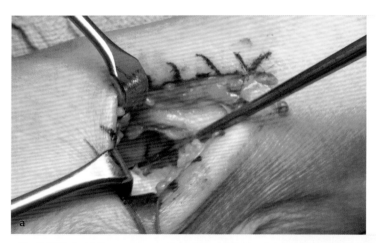
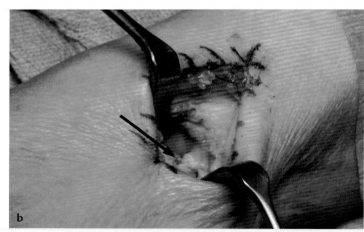

Fig. 2.154 (a,b) Suspension arthroplasty with the intra-articularly obtained FCRL. Alternatively, one-third of the APL tendon can be harvested without an additional incision, guided through the dorsal section of the capsule, and placed under the FCRL (arrow). It is fixed to the FCRL while the thumb is held under longitudinal tension, and then sutured again to itself.

Chapter 3

The Elbow

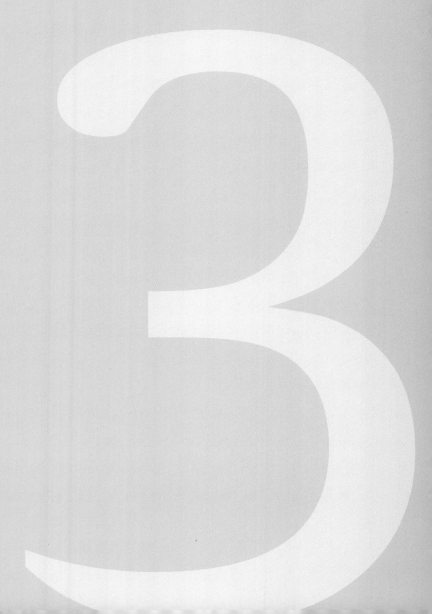

3 The Elbow

S. Sell, S. Rehart, C. Chan, M. Henniger

3.1 Elbow Synovectomy

3.1.1 Arthroscopic Synovectomy of the Elbow Joint

▶ **Indication.** Therapy-resistant Larsen 0–II/III synovitis after optimization of medication therapy and cortisone injections.

▶ **Specific disclosures for patient consent.** Recurrence. Infection. Nerve injury. Radiosynoviorthesis and/or chemosynoviorthesis may be necessary 6 weeks postoperatively.

▶ **Instruments.** Standard elbow arthroscope. Special item: shaver system. Electrocautery.

▶ **Position.** Supine. Tourniquet on the proximal upper arm. Suspend the arm using an arm traction device with the elbow joint in 90° of flexion (see ▶ Fig. 3.1).

▶ **Approach.** See ▶ Fig. 3.2, ▶ Fig. 3.3, ▶ Fig. 3.4, ▶ Fig. 3.5.

▶ **Surgical technique.** See ▶ Fig. 3.6.

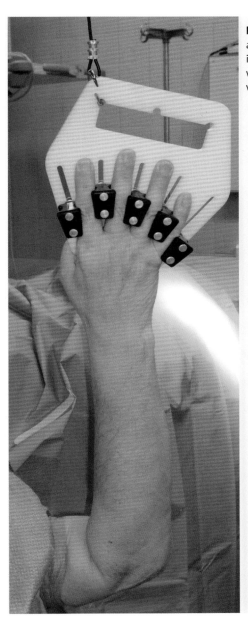

Fig. 3.1 Positioning and draping. The arm is in a traction device with a 3-kg counterweight on each side.

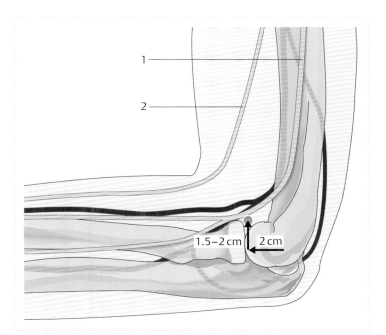

Fig. 3.2 Anterolateral approach: 2 cm distal and 1.5–2 cm anterior to the lateral epicondyle. 1, Radial nerve. 2, Lateral cutaneous nerve of forearm.

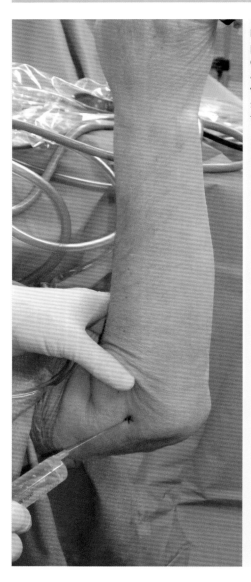

Fig. 3.3 The joint is punctured anterolateral to the radial head and synovial fluid is withdrawn for analysis. The joint is insufflated with fluid.

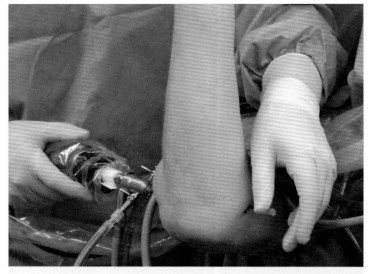

Fig. 3.4 Following insertion of the trocar and insufflation of the joint, the second portal is placed on the contralateral side under direct vision.

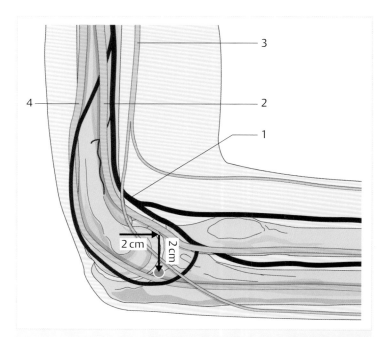

Fig. 3.5 Anteromedial approach: 2 cm distal and 2 cm anterior to the medial epicondyle. 1, Brachial artery. 2, Median nerve. 3, Medial cutaneous nerve of forearm. 4, Ulnar nerve.

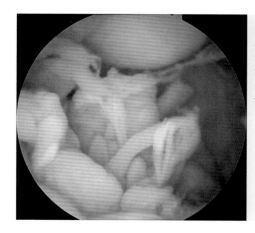

Fig. 3.6 Severe intra-articular elbow joint synovitis. Synovectomy is performed using a shaver and vaporizer.

3.1.2 Open Synovectomy of the Elbow Joint

▶ **Indication.** Therapy-resistant Larsen 0–II/III synovitis after optimization of medication therapy, cortisone injections, and, if indicated, arthroscopic synovectomy. Ultrasound evidence of loculated synovitis or extra-articular bursae/rheumatic nodules.

Significant clinical symptoms and loss of mobility, particularly a functional loss such as an extension deficit, are indications for an open procedure. Painful pronation/supination and radial head destruction are indications for radial head excision. Late synovectomy is also indicated for more advanced stages of destruction.

▶ **Specific disclosures for patient consent.** Recurrence. Infection. Loss of mobility with scarring.

▶ **Instruments.** Standard surgical pans.

▶ **Position.** Supine. Arm extended outward. Use an arm or hand table if necessary.

▶ **Approach.** See ▶ Fig. 3.7, ▶ Fig. 3.8, ▶ Fig. 3.9.

▶ **Specifics.** Assess the extent of synovitis preoperatively (is a dorsal incision also necessary?).

▶ **Surgical technique.** See ▶ Fig. 3.10, ▶ Fig. 3.11.

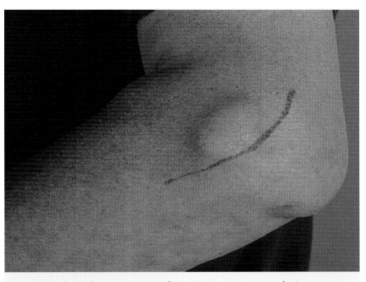

Fig. 3.7 A lateral incision is made starting approximately 3 cm proximal to the radial head and continued distally along the postero-lateral side of the radial head.

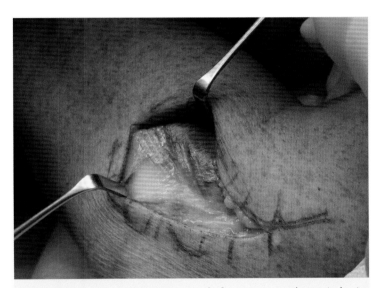

Fig. 3.8 The extensor digitorum muscle fascia is opened anteriorly. A strip of capsule approximately 1 cm wide is left on the humerus. A posterior opening is made in the fascia between the extensor carpi ulnaris muscle and the anconeus muscle. Musculature should not be detached from the humerus.

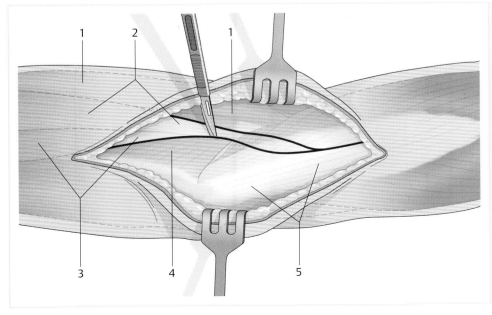

Fig. 3.9 Schematic drawing of the approach. An incision between the extensor carpi ulnaris and anconeus muscles exposes the posterior compartment. An incision between the extensor digitorum and the radial extensor muscles exposes the anterior compartment. 1, Extensor carpi radialis longus muscle. 2, Extensor digitorum muscle. 3, Extensor carpi ulnaris muscle. 4, Anconeus muscle. 5, Triceps brachii muscle tendon.

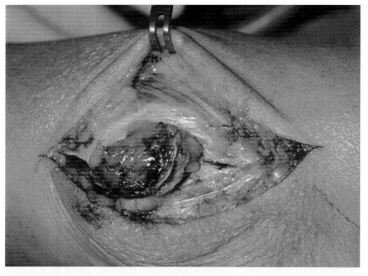

Fig. 3.10 Following posterior capsulotomy, bulging synovitis is readily apparent. View of the radial head. Synovectomy of the anterior compartment is performed with the elbow in flexion. The posterior compartment behind the retained muscle strip is more easily accessed with the elbow in extension. A posterior synovectomy is performed in the olecranon fossa. Caveat: the ulnar nerve lies relatively unprotected on the medial side.

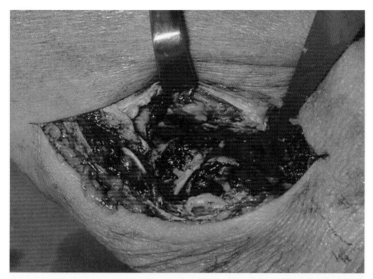

Fig. 3.11 Surgical site after open synovectomy. In case of a severe extension deficit, arthrolysis of the entire joint is also performed. The joint is easily accessible with the elbow in flexion. The capsule is released proximally from the humeral head and stripped off proximally approximately one hand's width from the joint. This is a safe distance from the radial nerve. If there is residual extensor deficit, the capsule is carefully incised on the coronoid process under direct vision. This incision is made from the top of the coronoid process, perpendicular to the axis of the ulna, and directed toward the midline. The capsule is stripped off with a rasp.

3.1.3 Resection of Rheumatic Nodules and Bursae in the Elbow

▶ **Indication.** Mechanically disruptive or enlarging rheumatic nodules accompanied by pronounced bursitis or acute olecranon bursitis. See also ▶ Fig. 3.12.

▶ **Specific disclosures for patient consent.** Impaired wound healing that may require secondary wound healing. Recurrence.

▶ **Instruments.** Standard surgical pans. Tourniquet.

▶ **Position.** Supine with arm stretched out on an arm table. If there is reduced mobility of the ipsilateral shoulder, then prone position with the arm freely hanging and flexed.

▶ **Surgical technique.** See ▶ Fig. 3.13.

▶ **Specific complications.** Impaired wound healing.

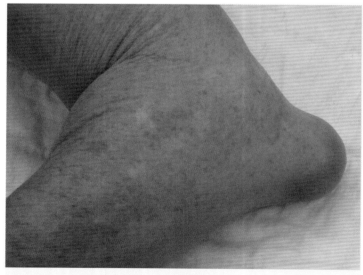

Fig. 3.12 Left elbow rheumatic nodule with concomitant olecranon bursitis. As a rule, a longitudinal skin incision is used because rheumatoid patients may need an elbow prosthesis later on.

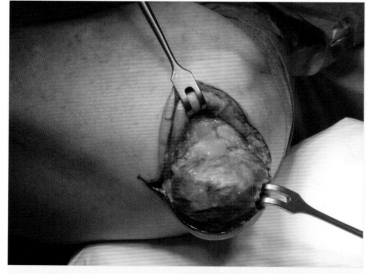

Fig. 3.13 View after extirpation of the rheumatic nodule and bursectomy. The ulnar nerve is identified

3.2 Elbow Prosthesis

▶ **Indication.** Larsen IV–V destruction. In situ destruction (bones/joints). Also for joints where the articular bony surfaces are still intact but functional stability has been lost.

▶ **Specific disclosures for patient consent.** Prosthesis loosening; dislocation. Bone fracture; perforation. Infection. Loss of mobility.

▶ **Instruments.** Prosthesis system from the manufacturer of choice.

▶ **Position.** Prone. Place a short lateral positioning roll under the upper arm. The position must allow the elbow to be flexed. Arrange for intraoperative radiography. See also ▶ Fig. 3.14.

▶ **Specifics.** Beware position-related anterior compression injury to the median nerve and injury to the ulnar nerve at the surgical site (hooks, scalpel). Swab for laboratory analysis if needed.

▶ **Approach.** Posterior over the elbow. The technique is either to split the triceps, or make a V-shaped triceps reflecting tendon pedicle that remains attached to the olecranon. See also ▶ Fig. 3.18.

▶ **Key steps.** Determine the humeral insertion site for the cutting guide. Adjust the tension of both prosthesis components using trial implants. Patiently and carefully connect the permanent prosthesis components.

Various prosthesis systems are available, and run the gamut from uncoupled to fully coupled with all types of coupling mechanisms. The type of prosthesis indicated is dependent upon the preoperative condition of the bone and, above all, the level of preexisting joint stability.

▶ **Surgical technique.** See ▶ Fig. 3.15, ▶ Fig. 3.16, ▶ Fig. 3.17, ▶ Fig. 3.19, ▶ Fig. 3.20, ▶ Fig. 3.21, ▶ Fig. 3.22, ▶ Fig. 3.23, ▶ Fig. 3.24, ▶ Fig. 3.25, ▶ Fig. 3.26, ▶ Fig. 3.27, ▶ Fig. 3.28, ▶ Fig. 3.29, ▶ Fig. 3.30, ▶ Fig. 3.31, ▶ Fig. 3.32, ▶ Fig. 3.33.

▶ **Specifics.** Prosthesis revision (▶ Fig. 3.34, ▶ Fig. 3.35).

▶ **Specific complications.** Beware the risk of creating a false passage while preparing the medullary canals. Osteoporotic bones are at risk for intraoperative fracture. Nerve injury.

▶ **Postoperative aftercare.** Immediate full-range mobilization. Initially, immobilize for 2 weeks in a plaster shell splint in 30° flexion. Wrap carefully at night and avoid excess tension on the suture line as this may lead to wound dehiscence and infection. Apply full active and passive range of motion for 20 minutes six times daily. See also ▶ Fig. 3.36.

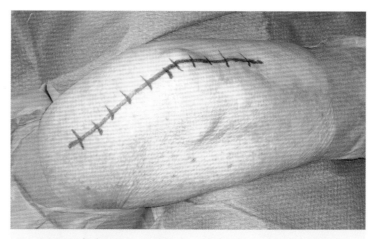

Fig. 3.14 With the patient in the lateral decubitus position, the elbow is draped freely over an arm support. The posterior skin incision is marked. The incision is longitudinal and curved slightly radially as needed.

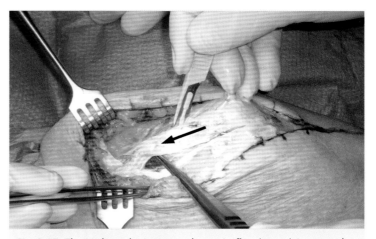

Fig. 3.15 The V-shaped triceps tendon strip flap (arrow) is created.

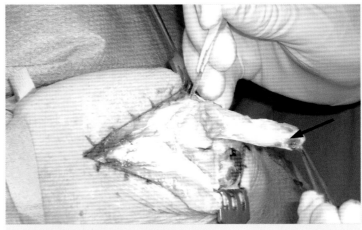

Fig. 3.16 The tendon strip pedicle is left attached to the olecranon (triceps tendon strip; arrow).

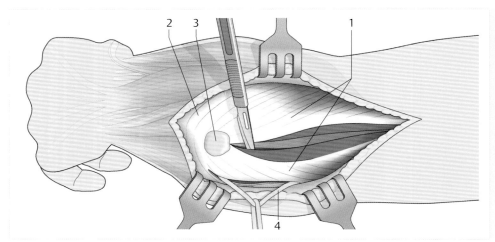

Fig. 3.18 Schematic drawing of the approach. 1, Triceps brachii muscle. 2, Extensor/flexor carpi ulnaris. 3, Olecranon. 4, Ulnar nerve.

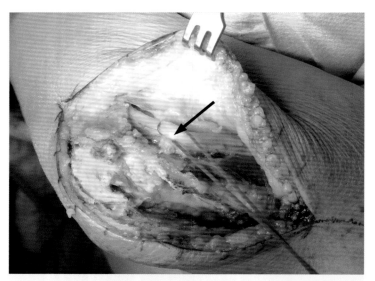

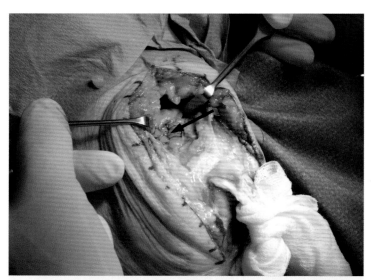

Fig. 3.17 An alternative approach is a longitudinal triceps split. Here the triceps is detached from the ulnar bone using an osteotome. The ulnar nerve (arrow), frequently with adhesions due to inflammation, is exposed and loop retracted. Retraction is particularly important with preexisting severe joint synovitis because the nerve lies unprotected next to the synovial tissue where the synovectomy is performed.

Fig. 3.19 Synovectomy of the posterior joint compartment. Synovitis in the olecranon fossa (arrow).

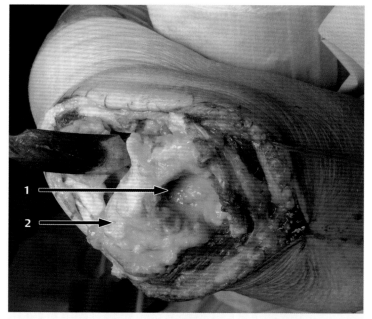

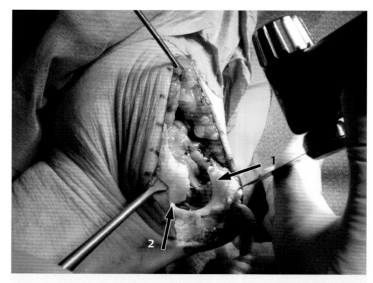

Fig. 3.20 The distal humerus is exposed. 1, Olecranon fossa. 2, Humeral condyles.

Fig. 3.21 The periarticular portion of the olecranon and its tip are resected (1). The tip of the coronoid process is excised and the capsule is detached from the coronoid process (2). An arthrolysis facilitates exposure of the joint.

3

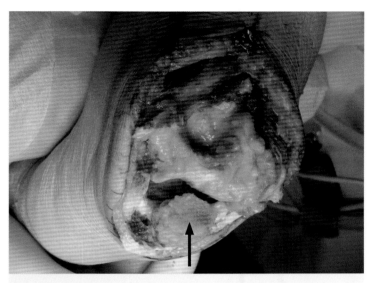

Fig. 3.22 Resection of the radial head (arrow) and synovectomy.

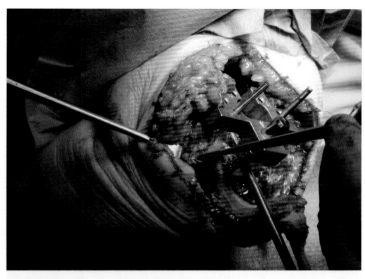

Fig. 3.23 The humeral shaft is opened and reamed. Caveat: proceed very carefully with osteoporotic bone. The resection and drill guide are attached for preparation of the distal humerus (GSB III Zimmer Biomet, Winterthur, Switzerland). The joint surfaces are resected.

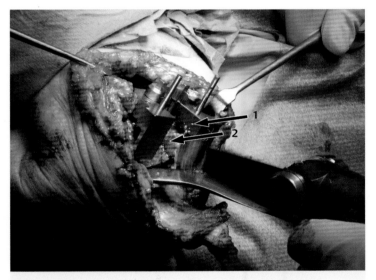

Fig. 3.24 The humeral box guide is positioned onto the distal humerus. Great care must be taken not to remove too much of the proximal medial and lateral epicondyles when performing the osteotomy within the box. 1, Box guide. 2, Intracondylar box osteotomy.

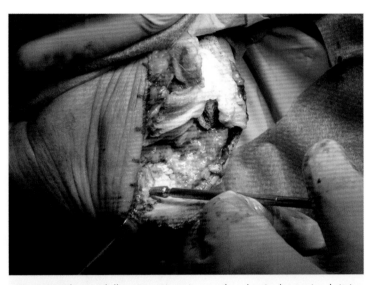

Fig. 3.25 The medullary insertion site on the ulna is determined. It is positioned far posterior. Reaming is done with medullary reamers of increasing sizes. The tissue is frequently very sclerosed.

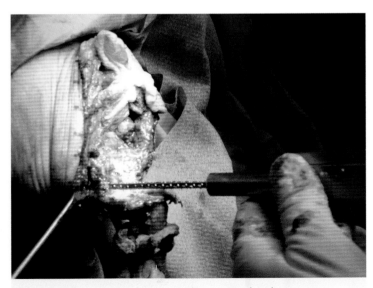

Fig. 3.26 The ulnar medullary canal is prepared with a rasp.

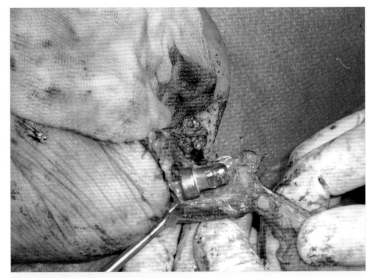

Fig. 3.27 The ulnar trial implant is inserted.

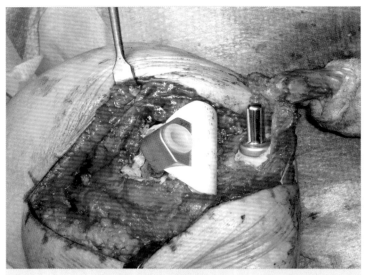

Fig. 3.28 Cemented placement of humeral and ulnar prosthesis components. A high-viscosity cement is recommended for better filling of the medullary canal due to its narrow size.

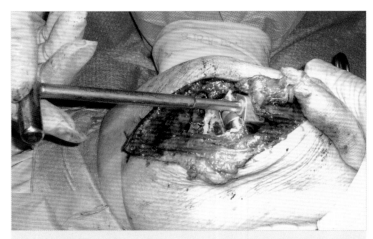

Fig. 3.29 The prosthesis components are carefully connected.

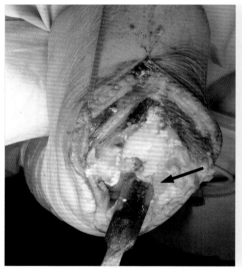

Fig. 3.30 A constrained prosthesis is inserted if there is significant joint instability. The prosthesis box and the medial and lateral epicondyles are carefully prepared. Arrow indicates the resected box.

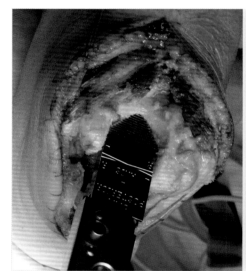

Fig. 3.31 The humeral shaft is prepared with a rasp.

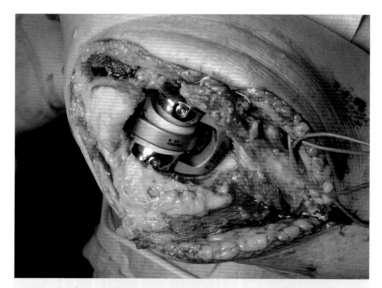

Fig. 3.32 The prosthesis components can be individually cemented first and then coupled. This facilitates later potential revisions. During insertion into the humeral canal, a piece of bone can be placed anteriorly under the prosthesis component, if needed.

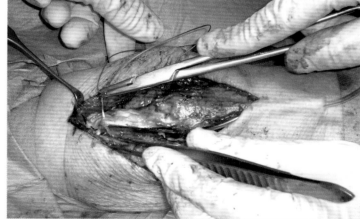

Fig. 3.33 The triceps brachii muscle tendon is repaired as part of the wound closure.

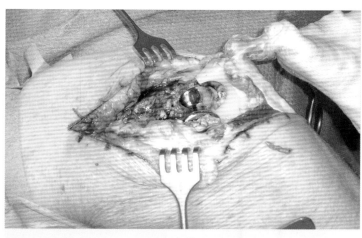

Fig. 3.34 Loosened unconstrained elbow prosthesis.

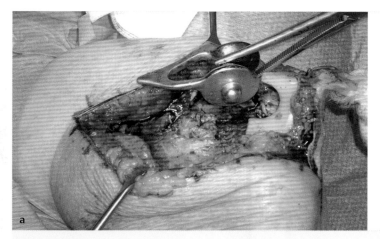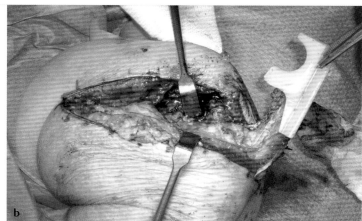

Fig. 3.35 (a,b) Explantation of the loosened Souter prosthesis.

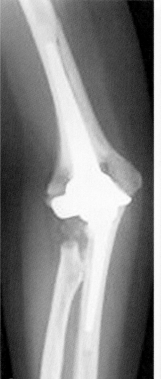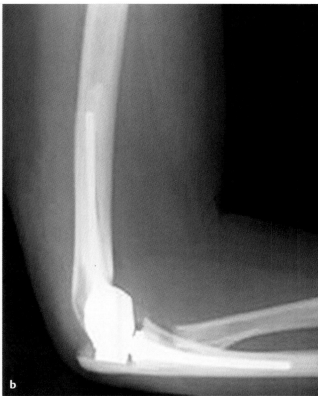

Fig. 3.36 (a,b) Postoperative radiographs of a GSB III prosthesis in situ.

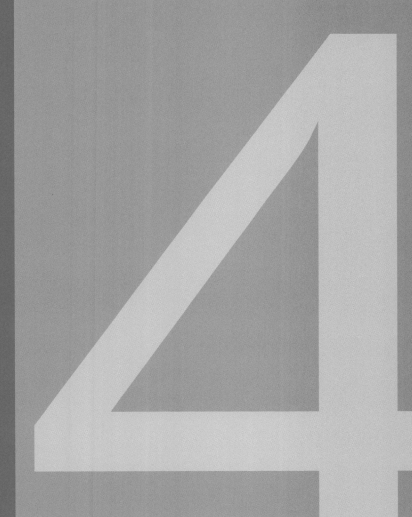

Chapter 4

The Shoulder

4 The Shoulder

S. Rehart, S. Sell, C. Chan, A. Sachs

4.1 Arthroscopic Synovectomy of the Shoulder Joint

▶ **Indication.** Therapy-resistant Larsen 0–II/III synovitis after optimization of medication therapy and cortisone injections. Significant clinical symptoms and loss of mobility.

▶ **Specific disclosures for patient consent.** Recurrence. Infection. Radiosynoviorthesis (and/or chemosynoviorthesis) may be necessary 6 weeks postoperatively.

▶ **Instruments.** Standard shoulder arthroscope. Special items: shaver system. Electrocautery.

▶ **Position.** Beach chair position with arm freely mobile (▶ Fig. 4.1).

▶ **Approach.** See ▶ Fig. 4.2, ▶ Fig. 4.3.

▶ **Specifics.** Preoperative ultrasound is used for evaluation of the major extra-articular bursae; these may necessitate an open procedure. Mark the anatomical landmarks (acromion, coracoid, scapular border, clavicle) after sterile draping and prior to making an incision.

▶ **Surgical technique.** See ▶ Fig. 4.4, ▶ Fig. 4.5, ▶ Fig. 4.6, ▶ Fig. 4.7, ▶ Fig. 4.8, ▶ Fig. 4.9.

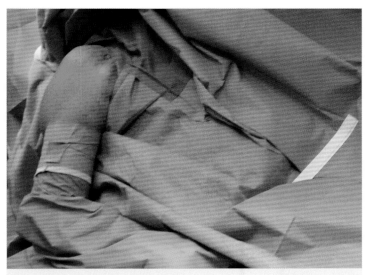

Fig. 4.1 Positioning and draping.

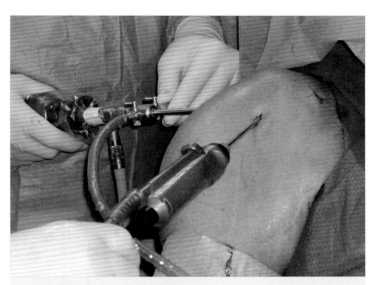

Fig. 4.3 The standard approach is from posterior. Instrument (here a shaver) from anterior.

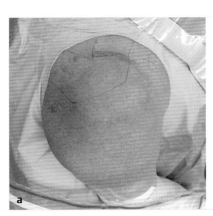
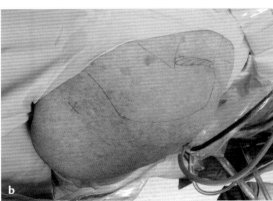

Fig. 4.2 (a,b) The anatomical structures and standard arthroscopic portal sites are marked. The posterior humeral head is palpated. The capsule is bluntly penetrated following a stab incision placed 1 cm inferior and medial to the lateral tip of the acromion. The anterior portal is placed under direct arthroscopic vision.

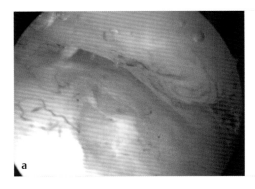

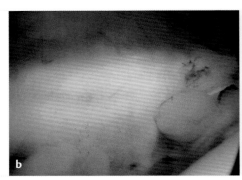

Fig. 4.4 (a,b) Intra-articular synovitis.

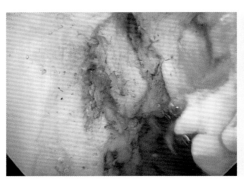

Fig. 4.5 Synovectomy is performed using a vaporizer, particularly for severe inflammatory processes, due to improved hemostasis.

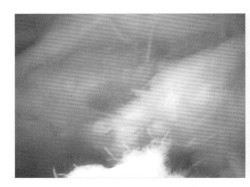

Fig. 4.6 Pronounced rotator cuff tear.

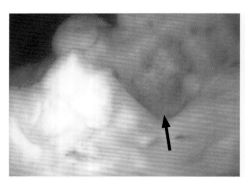

Fig. 4.7 Synovitis-induced bone defect with erosion on the humeral head (arrow).

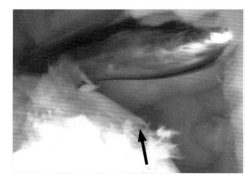

Fig. 4.8 Significant cartilage damage is readily apparent (arrow).

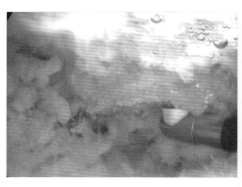

Fig. 4.9 Subacromial decompression may be required. Bone should be removed judiciously and only where needed. The synovitis is completely removed, and the area is cauterized with the vaporizer. Radiosynoviorthesis is scheduled 6 to 8 weeks later.

4.2 Rotator Cuff Tear

▶ **Indication.** Larsen I–II destruction. Rotator cuff tear diagnosed by radiographic imaging (MRI scan, ultrasound).

Operatively reconstructible rotator cuff tear: based on size on MRI scan and no evidence of fatty degeneration of musculature on MRI scan. Acromiohumeral interval greater than 6 mm.

If there is any uncertainty, rotator cuff mobility can be examined arthroscopically.

▶ **Specific disclosures for patient consent.** Failure of tendon integration. Re-rupture (also secondarily with cranialization of the humeral head). Shoulder stiffness. Injury to blood vessels, nerves (for example, axillary nerve).

▶ **Instruments.** Standard shoulder arthroscopy pan. Shoulder pan. Anchoring system from the manufacturer of choice.

▶ **Position.** Beach chair position (▶ Fig. 4.10).

▶ **Key steps.** Proceed in the same fashion as for shoulder arthroscopy. Every rheumatoid shoulder first undergoes arthroscopy, see Chapter 4.1.

Synovectomy is initially performed arthroscopically on each patient. The inflamed bursa is removed during the subsequent subacromial arthroscopy. Rotator cuff mobility is assessed. Small ruptures are closed arthroscopically, although these are relatively uncommon in rheumatoid patients. The quality of the rotator cuff tissue surrounding the rupture is frequently poor and is usually associated with severe subacromial inflammatory changes. As a result, a mini-open approach is often chosen.

▶ **Surgical technique.** See ▶ Fig. 4.11, ▶ Fig. 4.12, ▶ Fig. 4.13, ▶ Fig. 4.14, ▶ Fig. 4.15, ▶ Fig. 4.16, ▶ Fig. 4.17, ▶ Fig. 4.18.

▶ **Postoperative aftercare.** Immediate full-range mobilization (caveat: no shoulder immobilization). For large ruptures, use a shoulder abduction pillow for 6 weeks.

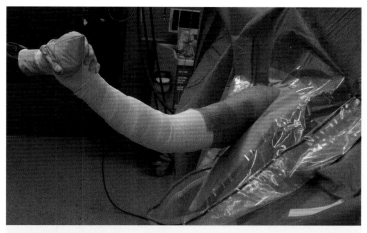

Fig. 4.10 The shoulder with the patient placed in the beach chair position.

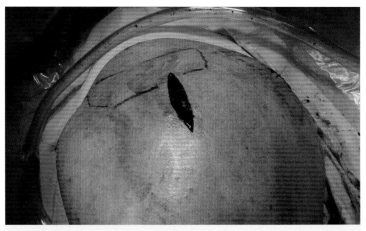

Fig. 4.11 The rotator cuff is evaluated arthroscopically to determine reparability. A longitudinal skin incision is made starting at the acromial edge and extending 2 to 3 cm distally along the direction of the deltoid muscle fibers. The deltoid muscle fibers are split longitudinally, and a spreader is inserted.

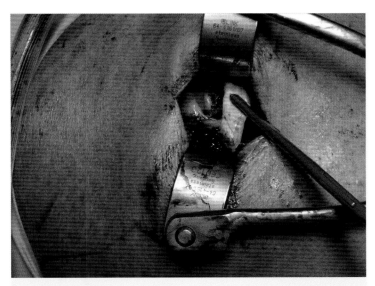

Fig. 4.12 The biceps tendon (forceps) is clearly dislocated and severely damaged due to the large rupture. The tendon is tenotomized, but a fixation is typically avoided.

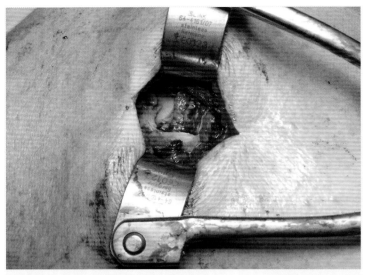

Fig. 4.13 The rotator cuff tear also extends centrally to the lower acromial edge. The inflammatory tissue is removed, and the edges are debrided. The rupture is extensively mobilized.

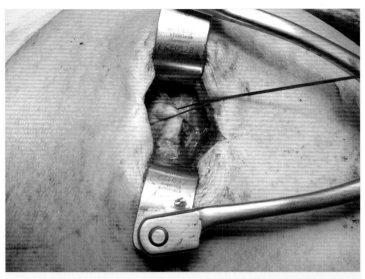

Fig. 4.14 A stay suture is placed around the rupture for mobilization.

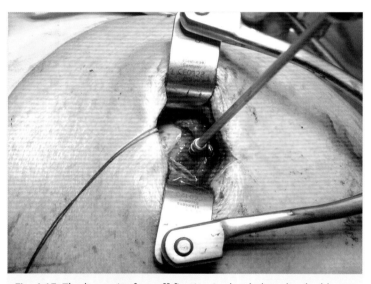

Fig. 4.15 The bone site for cuff fixation is abraded, and a double-loaded suture anchor is inserted.

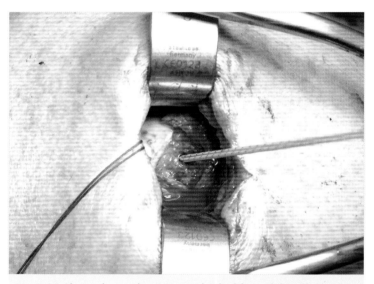

Fig. 4.16 The anchor and suture are checked for stability (the bone is frequently very osteoporotic).

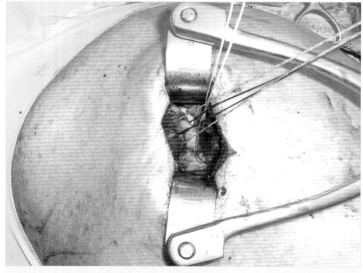

Fig. 4.17 The cuff is grasped with a Mason–Allen stitch. It is fixed with the anchor sutures and then side-to-side closure is completed.

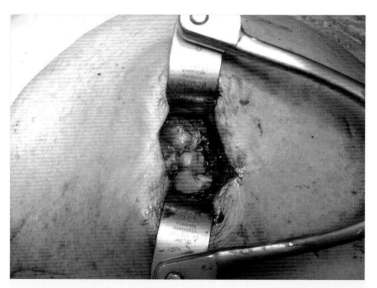

Fig. 4.18 Fully reconstructed tear.

4.3 Shoulder Endoprosthesis

4.3.1 Head Resurfacing/Head Replacement

The indications for the various prostheses are based on the amount of bone destruction. However, the condition of the rotator cuff is the primary consideration.

A deliberate decision has been made not to depict here an anatomical shoulder prosthesis system. The preparation and placement of a socket and shaft are described in the reverse total shoulder prosthesis section (Chapter 4.3.2).

▶ **Indication.** Larsen III–V destruction with humeral head destruction and significant clinical symptoms. No large rotator cuff tear. A socket without major destruction and a centered humeral head. Shoulders that have considerable fatty degeneration of the rotator cuff (on MRI scan) or severe osteoporosis/humeral head necrosis are not suitable for a surface replacement arthroplasty. A surface replacement is usually performed without implanting a socket.

Humeral head replacement is an option for humeral head necrosis, which frequently occurs in rheumatoid illnesses.

▶ **Specific disclosures for patient consent.** Prosthesis loosening, dislocation. Tendon rupture (also secondary). Bone fracture, perforation. Damage to sensory nerve branches. Nerve injuries (axillary nerve).

▶ **Instruments.** Prosthesis system from the manufacturer of choice.

▶ **Position.** Beach chair position. Radiography must be available! Ensure that the arm can be fully extended.

▶ **Approach.** Deltopectoral approach. See also ▶ Fig. 4.19.

▶ **Key steps.** Protect the axillary nerve (from retractor compression, for example). Perform a subacromial bursa resection if necessary. Leave approximately 5 mm of subscapular tendon on the lesser tuberosity for subsequent refixation. Alternatively, release the scapularis muscle by performing an osteotomy of the bone. Precise placement of the alignment guide for the head resection is important.

▶ **Surgical technique.** See ▶ Fig. 4.20, ▶ Fig. 4.21, ▶ Fig. 4.22, ▶ Fig. 4.23, ▶ Fig. 4.24, ▶ Fig. 4.25, ▶ Fig. 4.26, ▶ Fig. 4.27, ▶ Fig. 4.28, ▶ Fig. 4.29, ▶ Fig. 4.30.

▶ **Specific complications.** Failed subscapularis muscle suture repair. Axillary nerve injury.

▶ **Postoperative aftercare.** Immediate full-range mobilization. Gilchrist bandage for 2 days, then an abduction pillow for 3 weeks. Initially passive mobilization to 70° abduction, 10° external rotation, 90° anteversion. Active assisted mobilization from the third week on. Early finger exercise.

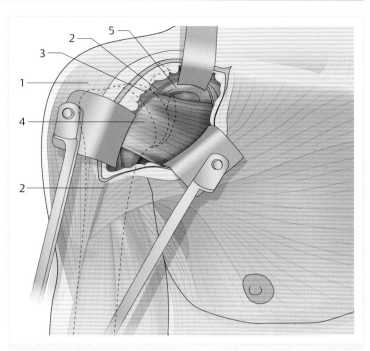

Fig. 4.19 Schematic drawing of the approach. This approach allows for plenty of options to extend the incision in the event of intraoperative complications, such as fracture. 1, Deltoid muscle. 2, Cephalic vein. 3, Short head of biceps brachii muscle. 4, Subscapularis muscle. 5, Coracoid process.

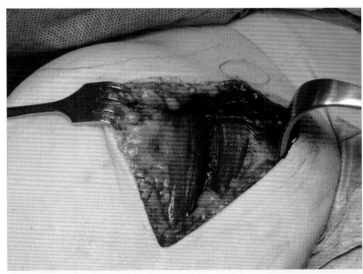

Fig. 4.20 A skin incision is made starting at the coracoid process (marked) and extended along the deltopectoral groove. The tissue is dissected down to the deltopectoral groove. The groove is bluntly dissected. The cephalic vein and the deltoid muscle fibers are together retracted laterally.

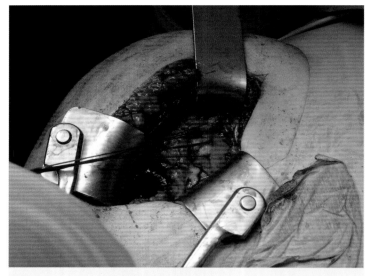

Fig. 4.21 The subscapularis muscle tendon is looped with a minimum of three retaining sutures. A tendon strip at least 5 mm wide is left on the humeral head for subsequent refixation. Alternative: release the tendon from the humerus with a fleck osteotomy (use caution with osteoporotic bone).

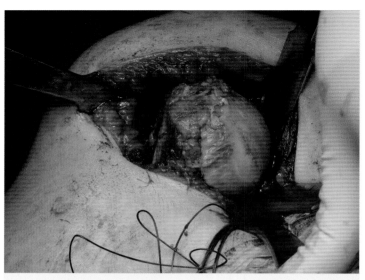

Fig. 4.22 Mobilization of the humeral head. All osteophytes are removed, and the capsule is released from the humeral head. The pectoral muscle is incised if there is contracture with poor external rotation.

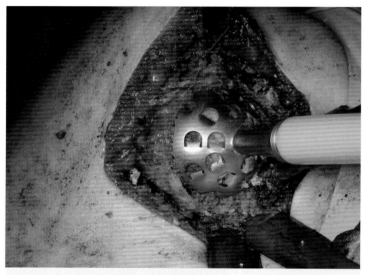

Fig. 4.23 The guidewire is inserted into the center of the humerus using a template sizer. When selecting the appropriate head size (radiographic templating), avoid using a head that is too large since it may "overstuff" the joint. The template is fitted to precisely match the bone edges of the humeral head. The line where cartilage meets bone allows for precise three-dimensional alignment of the reamer template with the patient's native anatomy. Humeral head shaping and débridement is performed over the guidewire.

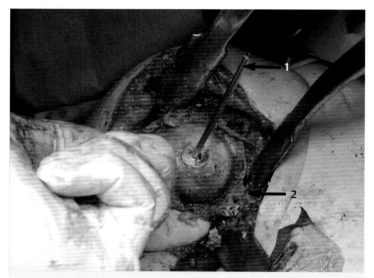

Fig. 4.24 The central alignment pin (1) is prepared over the central guidewire. Bone spurs are excised (2).

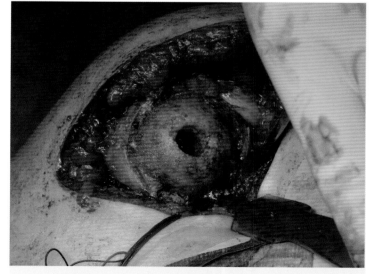

Fig. 4.25 The humeral head is finally prepared by drilling the central anchorage hole.

4

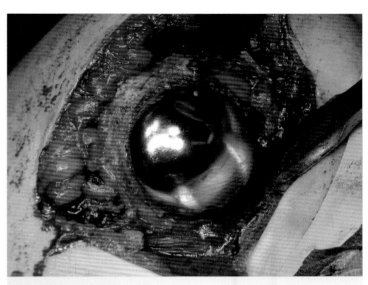

Fig. 4.26 Final metal implant.

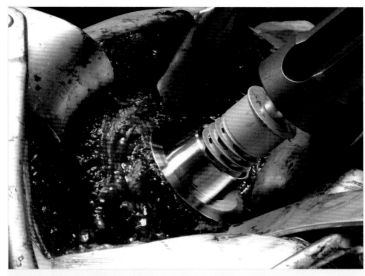

Fig. 4.28 Insertion of the central anchoring screw.

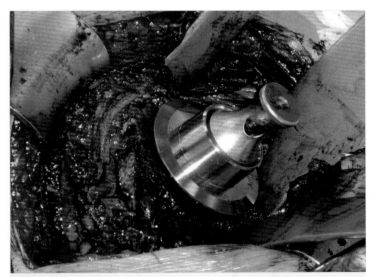

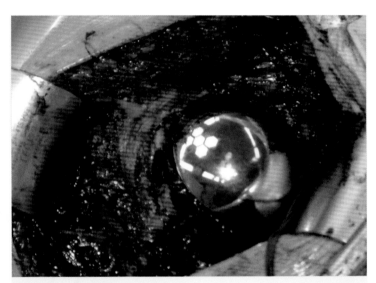

Fig. 4.29 Impacted permanent metal implant.

Fig. 4.27 Humeral head replacement is an option for preexisting humeral head necrosis with sufficient remaining humeral bone quality. The humeral head is osteotomized at the cartilage/metaphyseal border, which is easily exposed following removal of all osteophytes. The natural retroversion of the humeral head can thus be maintained. This is also a better option in the event of a socket replacement, and is definitely beneficial for rheumatoid patients who still have an intact rotator cuff. In case of an isolated head surface replacement a glenoid component can be considerably difficult.

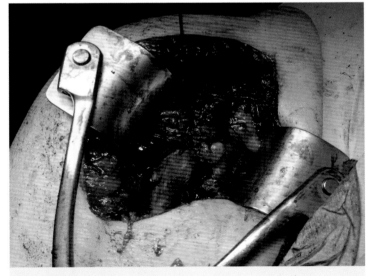

Fig. 4.30 The cuff and subscapularis muscle are repaired using Mason–Allen stitches.

4.3.2 Reverse Shoulder Prosthesis

This procedure requires extensive experience in the operative care of the shoulder. It is often difficult to expose the glenoid.

▶ **Indication.** Nonreparable rotator cuff lesions with Larsen IV–V joint destruction and significant clinical symptoms. Age greater than 65 years, because revision is difficult in those patients.

▶ **Specific disclosures for patient consent.** Prosthesis loosening, dislocation. Loss of shoulder function. Bone fracture, perforation. Scapular notching. Rocking-horse phenomenon.

▶ **Instruments.** Prosthesis system from manufacturer of choice.

▶ **Position.** Beach chair position. Fluoroscopy must be available.

▶ **Specifics.** The shaft can be implanted cemented or uncemented. The convex component of the total prosthesis system is fixed to the glenoid (center of rotation is moved medially and distally). Shoulder mobility is now primarily dependent on deltoid muscle movement. Preoperative MRI/CT imaging is recommended to properly assess glenoid orientation. Neurological evaluation of the axillary nerve is mandatory for a reoperation on the affected shoulder.

▶ **Approach.** Deltopectoral; alternatively, superior-lateral (McKenzie approach).

▶ **Key steps.** Orientation of the prepared humeral guides and preparation of the socket (precise orientation of the metaglene!). Note: precise placement of the glenoid screw is important. It is essential to perform the trial implant reduction under appropriate tension.

The approach is the same as for humeral head surface arthroplasty of the shoulder (see Chapter 4.3.1).

▶ **Surgical technique.** See ▶ Fig. 4.31, ▶ Fig. 4.32, ▶ Fig. 4.33, ▶ Fig. 4.34, ▶ Fig. 4.35, ▶ Fig. 4.36, ▶ Fig. 4.37, ▶ Fig. 4.38, ▶ Fig. 4.39.

▶ **Specific complications.** Notching. Rocking. Loss of motion. (Sub-)Luxation. Axillary nerve injury.

▶ **Postoperative aftercare.** Immediate full-range mobilization.

For 6 weeks, passive abduction and 90° anteversion with careful external and internal rotation. No weight-supporting movements. Use an abduction pillow if needed (to relieve tension on the deltoid muscle), then gradually increase to unrestricted activity.

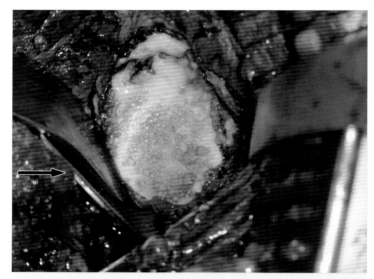

Fig. 4.31 The destroyed socket is exposed. Extensive capsular release (periosteal) is frequently necessary both on the shaft and circumferentially around the socket. Following osteotomy of the humeral head, a humeral stem protector (arrow) is placed to prevent injury from retractor pressure.

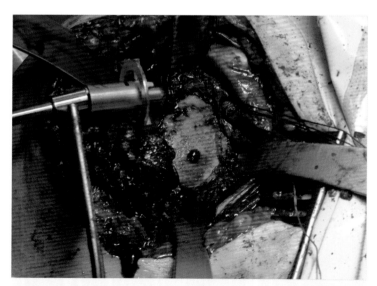

Fig. 4.32 Preparation of the glenoid is performed according to the surgical instructions provided by the manufacturer of the specific prosthesis system. It is important to accurately determine the entry point into the socket. Preoperative CT imaging provides information regarding the location of maximal socket wear and any necessary correction of the reamer orientation needed to achieve a flat support surface.

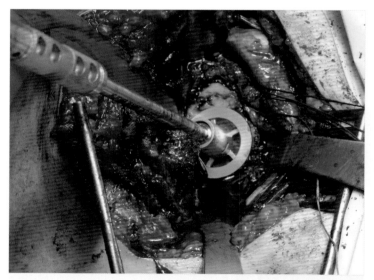

Fig. 4.33 The sclerotic sections of the glenoid are debrided. The socket position is very important in order to prevent later scapular notching (from the humeral cup rim).

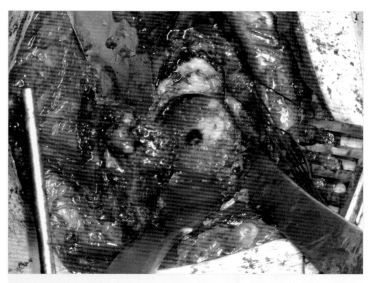

Fig. 4.34 View of the prepared glenoid surface.

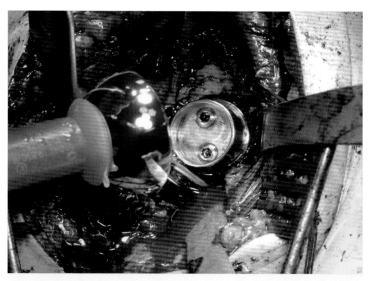

Fig. 4.35 Surgical site with base plate prior to metaglene placement.

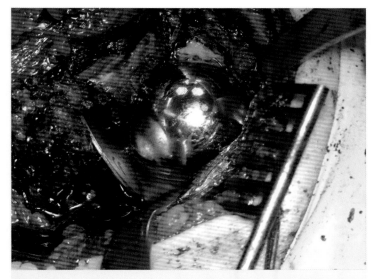

Fig. 4.36 In situ position of the metaglene. The humerus with stem protector is to the left.

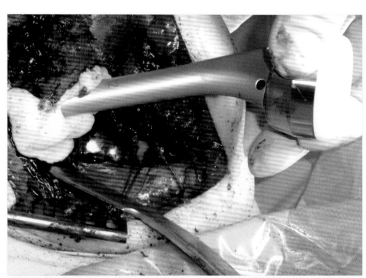

Fig. 4.37 Cemented insertion of the humerus shaft following humeral reaming.

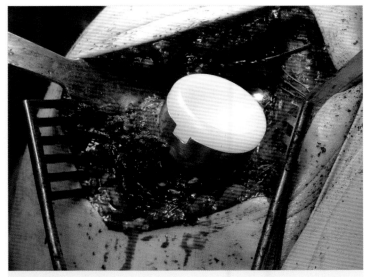

Fig. 4.38 Position after insertion of the cemented humerus shaft and liner.

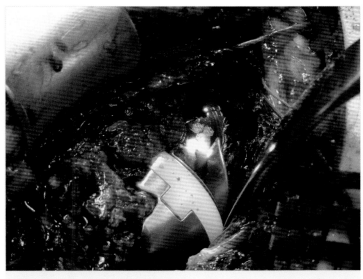

Fig. 4.39 Prosthesis components are reduced under optimal tension.

Chapter 5

The Foot

5 The Foot

S. Sell, S. Rehart, M. Henniger, B. Kurosch

5.1 Indications and Therapeutic Plan

In 85 to 90% of rheumatoid patients the foot is affected, to some extent also early in the disease process. The forefoot is most commonly involved, followed by the midfoot and ankle joint.

The fundamental principle of therapy—proximal before distal—also applies to the foot. Thus, lower ankle joint destruction should be addressed before treating forefoot involvement. It is, however, essential to keep in mind that every rheumatic patient requires an individual approach.

Forefoot synovectomies are rarely performed. In addition, joint-preserving procedures are becoming increasingly prevalent. The key factor in determining indications for treatment, more so than for the nonrheumatoid forefoot, is the condition of the soft tissues. On the one hand, the inflammatory process can lead to soft tissue contractures that can only be partially corrected. This plays a far greater role than the existence of bony deformities when determining indications for a joint-preservation intervention. If, for example, the great toe proximal joint is no longer reducible into a neutral position preoperatively, we believe there is tremendously increased risk of recurrence and that it is worth considering whether an arthrodesis would not be more advantageous. This is even more of a consideration if the great toe deformity has led to a fibular deviation of the second through fifth toes. The focus, therefore, should be on stabilizing and correcting the first ray.

On the other hand, the condition of the medial capsule plays a significant role in determining indications for treatment. The capsule structures are sometimes extremely elongated in rheumatoid patients and can lead to recurrence despite a good bony corrective result. It is, however, often quite difficult to evaluate the condition of the medial capsule preoperatively. Because of this, we have a frank discussion with these patients and inform them that the final decision between joint preservation or fusion will be determined intraoperatively, depending upon the soft tissues.

On the whole, the second through fifth toes are more difficult to correct than the great toes, which is an important consideration when determining the course of treatment.

Toe deformities are frequently associated with additional anatomical changes:
- Extensor tendon contractures (consider extensor tendon elongation).
- Dislocation of proximal joints (consider joint arthrolysis or a Weil osteotomy with dorsal wedge).
- Lateral elongation of the capsule with fibular deviation of the toes (consider capsuloplasty and duplication).

Despite the emergence of joint-preserving operations, forefoot metatarsal head resection continues to remain the "gold standard." It is also one of the "number one" procedures, because it is as successful and subjectively satisfying for the patient as the hip and knee prosthesis. We also favor this procedure at the outset of the surgical intervention plan outlined for the patients. The procedure can be performed from either a dorsal or a plantar approach, depending upon the surgeon's training; both procedures presented here produce good results. It is not unusual to perform bilateral forefoot corrections in order to minimize hospitalizations.

Arthrodesis is the standard procedure for correction of the first ray in the presence of contracture. A Swanson prosthesis presents an alternative for joint destruction with correctable soft tissue.

Because the soft tissue has a pivotal role in both indications and the operative approach, it should be protected during the postoperative healing process by use of orthotics or individually fitted ergonomic equipment.

Impaired wound healing is a major issue for rheumatoid patients due to the underlying illness and its associated medication therapy.

5.2 Proximal Corrective Osteotomy

▶ **Indication.** Severe rheumatic splayfoot. Rheumatic splayfoot with an intermetatarsal angle ≥ 18°. Soft tissues must be correctable. Larsen I–II destruction.

▶ **Specific disclosures for patient consent.** Impaired wound healing. Pseudarthrosis. Metatarsal head necrosis with sequelae (arthrodesis). Joint stiffness. Recurrence. Infection. Tendon injury. Blood vessel, nerve injury.

▶ **Instruments.** Locking plate. For L-shaped or Z-shaped screw fixation osteosynthesis, 2.7 to 4.0-mm cancellous screws.

▶ **Position.** Supine. Foot in neutral position with toes pointed upward. A pelvic support and tilting of the table can be used to achieve a better ankle position. Lower the contralateral foot. The foot is positioned with the edge of the heel over the end of the table.

Intraoperative radiographic imaging is only rarely needed.

▶ **Key steps.** An intermetatarsal skin incision is made between the first and second toes to repair soft tissues: release the adductor hallucis muscle and, depending upon the specific situation, perform a lateral release (see Chapter 5.3).

▶ **Surgical technique.** See ▶ Fig. 5.1, ▶ Fig. 5.2, ▶ Fig. 5.3, ▶ Fig. 5.4, ▶ Fig. 5.5.
Alternative: crescentic osteotomy at the first metatarsal base.

▶ **Postoperative aftercare.** An orthotic to protect the soft tissues is worn full time for 6 weeks, and then at nighttime only for an additional 6 weeks. A forefoot decompression shoe is used for 6 weeks. After that, radiographic imaging is performed for clearance to full weight bearing. Soft cushion insoles are used after foot swelling has subsided.

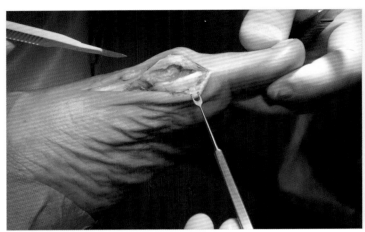

Fig. 5.1 A longitudinal skin incision is made starting at the base of the first metatarsal and continued to the first metatarsophalangeal joint. The capsule is split longitudinally. Alternatively, two separate skin incisions can be made: a longitudinal 3-cm incision placed more dorsally, starting at the base of the first metatarsal, and the same incision placed more proximally on the first metatarsophalangeal joint. Since we have not found that smaller incisions reduce wound healing complications, we frequently prefer a longer incision for improved exposure. The dorsomedial neurovascular bundle is exposed. The sensory cutaneous nerve runs from dorsal to plantar, and crosses over the distal end of the more longitudinally oriented vessel.

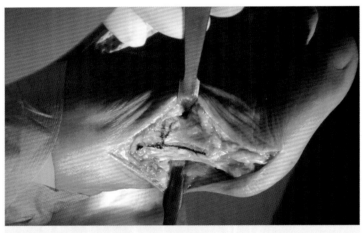

Fig. 5.2 The first metatarsal shaft axis and the predetermined proximal osteotomy planes are marked. A closing wedge osteotomy plane has been drawn here. A similar approach is followed for an L-shaped osteotomy with screw fixation osteosynthesis. A proximal short Z-shaped osteotomy is also an alternative.

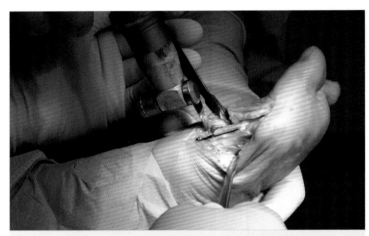

Fig. 5.3 The osteotomy is performed using two Hohmann elevators for protection. In the open-wedge technique, the lateral cortex remains intact. The osteotomy is then opened with two osteotomy chisels, taking care to preserve the integrity of the lateral cortex.

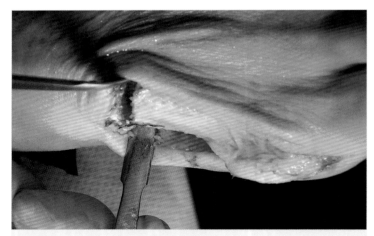

Fig. 5.4 The osteotomy edges are open. The amount of correction needed is determined from preoperative imaging and then implemented operatively. If needed, temporary K-wire fixation can be implemented to control instability or if the bone is very osteoporotic.

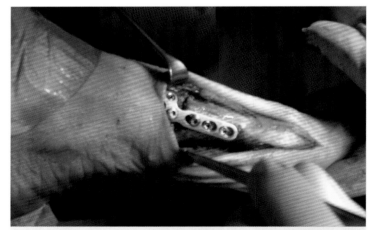

Fig. 5.5 Fixation is accomplished with a locking plate (plantar system as well if needed). The osteotomy gap width should remain uniform from dorsal to plantar. Plantarization of the first metatarsal base can be achieved by keeping the dorsal gap larger. A simultaneous soft tissue procedure is performed on the medial side of the proximal joint capsule apparatus.

5.3 Scarf Osteotomy

▶ **Indication.** Severe rheumatic splayfoot. Rheumatoid hallux valgus with an intermetatarsal angle of 10 to 18° (20°). Soft tissues must be correctable. Larsen I–II destruction.

▶ **Specific disclosures for patient consent.** Impaired wound healing. Pseudarthrosis. Metatarsal head necrosis with sequelae (arthrodesis). Recurrence. Infection. Joint stiffness. Tendon injury. Blood vessel, nerve injury.

Prosthesis placement is no longer possible following a Scarf osteotomy.

▶ **Instruments.** Screw 2.3-mm or 2.7-mm with flat head. Specialized countersinkable headless screws equipped with two different threads ("Herbert" screw).

▶ **Position.** Supine. Foot in neutral position with toes pointing upward. A pelvic support and tilting of the table can be used to achieve a better ankle position. Lower the contralateral foot. The foot is positioned with the edge of the heel over the end of the table.

Intraoperative radiographic imaging is only rarely needed.

▶ **Approach.** See ▶ Fig. 5.6, ▶ Fig. 5.7.

▶ **Surgical technique.** See ▶ Fig. 5.8, ▶ Fig. 5.9, ▶ Fig. 5.10, ▶ Fig. 5.11, ▶ Fig. 5.12, ▶ Fig. 5.13, ▶ Fig. 5.14.

▶ **Postoperative aftercare.** An orthotic to protect the soft tissues is worn full time for 6 weeks, and then at nighttime only for an additional 6 weeks. A forefoot decompression shoe is used for 6 weeks. After that, radiographic imaging is performed for clearance to full weight bearing. Soft cushion insoles are used once foot swelling has subsided.

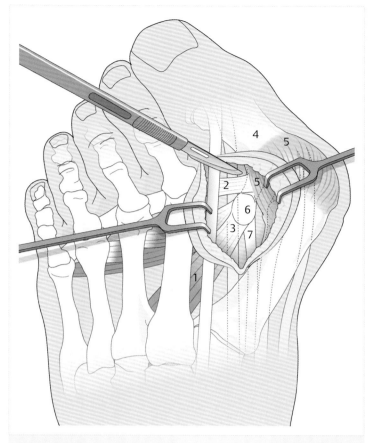

Fig. 5.7 Schematic drawing of the approach. The incision is made directly over the first metatarsal, where the risk of bleeding is lower. Blunt tissue dissection is performed down to the adductor hallucis muscle. The muscle is exposed and, if necessary, tenotomized after passing a clamp underneath. The lateral sesamoid bone is exposed (after palpation). The bone is detached and the lateral release is completed using a longitudinal incision. This must be reducible under the metatarsal head using light pressure. The release is terminated when the proximal joint is easily reducible into the desired position. If this cannot be achieved, the lateral joint capsule is weakened with multiple stab incisions. Forceful manipulation is used to achieve the desired position. 1, Adductor hallucis muscle. 2, Transverse metatarsal ligament. 3, Adductor hallucis tendon. 4, Proximal phalanx. 5, Great toe MTP joint capsule. 6, Fibular sesamoid bone. 7, Flexor hallucis brevis muscle.

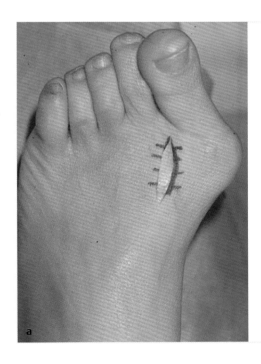
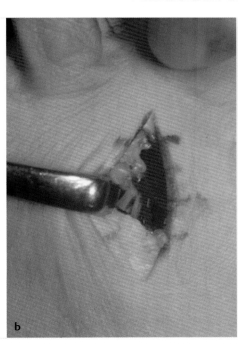

Fig. 5.6 (a,b) A longitudinal or **S**-shaped skin incision is made. An **S**-shaped incision curved toward the second metatarsal is recommended for a simultaneous procedure on the second MTP joint. Meticulous hemostasis is necessary because pronounced venous plexuses are frequently present.

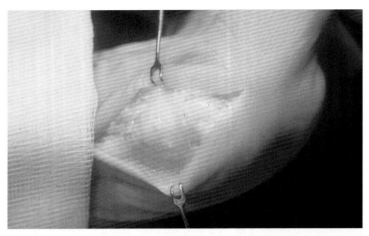

Fig. 5.8 The capsule and dorsomedial neurovascular bundle are exposed. The sensory cutaneous nerve runs from dorsal to plantar, and crosses over the distal end of the more longitudinally oriented vessel. A standard longitudinal capsulotomy is performed. An **L**-shaped capsulotomy is used only for pronounced deformities.

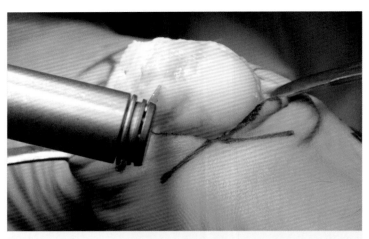

Fig. 5.9 The first metatarsal head is exposed following capsulotomy, and the inflamed tissue is synovectomized. The pseudoexostosis is osteotomized in a direction tangential to the axis of the shaft. The gutter border must be preserved because there is a small risk of varus deformity.

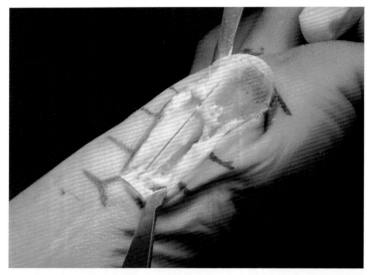

Fig. 5.10 A horizontal osteotomy of the first metatarsal base is completed from the proximal third of the plantar side of the shaft to the distal third of the dorsal aspect. The osteotomy cut is made with the saw aimed toward the fourth metatarsal. If a plantarization is also planned to treat particularly severe second-digit metatarsalgia, the osteotomy plane is sloped slightly toward plantar.

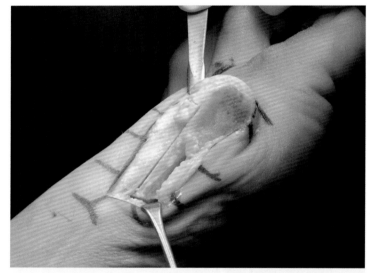

Fig. 5.11 The final proximal and distal cuts are made at an angle of approximately 60°. This leads to a better wedge and increased stability of the osteotomy fragments. The orientation of the proximal and distal osteotomies determines the lengthening (medial closing) or shortening (medial opening) of the first metatarsal needed to achieve the preoperative surgical goals.

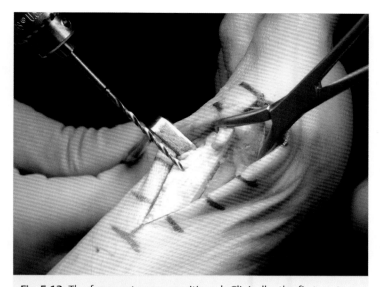

Fig. 5.12 The fragments are repositioned. Clinically, the first meta-tarsal head should come into direct contact with the second metatarsal head. This is rechecked by placing stress on the foot (forced splayfoot). As a rule, a 1-mm correction corresponds to a 1° change in the intermetatarsal angle. The metatarsal head is corrected by rotating the distal end of the fragment. We screw the fragments together with three 2.3-mm flat-head screws.

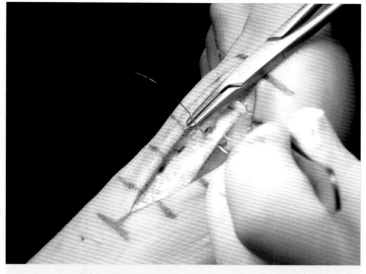

Fig. 5.14 Medial capsuloplasty. The capsular tissue is frequently very elongated in rheumatoid patients. In these cases we insert a 1.1-mm interosseous anchoring hole. It is advisable to grasp the capsule distally with a special suture technique. A Mason–Allen stitch, routinely used in shoulder surgery, is quite effective. The technique involves placing a transverse stitch through the capsule. A second stitch, placed longitudinally, anchors the suture. The capsule is then closed completely.

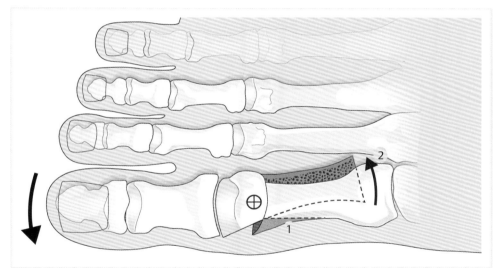

Fig. 5.13 Schematic drawing of the translation of the osteotomy surfaces.
The degree of lateral translation is determined by the intermetatarsal angle (1 mm translation corresponds to approximately 1° of correction) (1).
The distal metatarsal-articular angle (DMAA) is determined clinically. Rotation of the fragments (2) corrects the DMAA. This can be inspected clinically after repositioning.

5.4 Great Toe Metatarsophalangeal Joint Arthrodesis

▶ **Indication.** Larsen III–V great toe proximal joint destruction with significant clinical symptoms. Contracted hallux deformity (varus or valgus), not passively correctable, with severe rheumatic splayfoot (▶ Fig. 5.15).

▶ **Specific disclosures for patient consent.** Impaired wound healing. Pseudarthrosis. Infection. Tendon injury. Injury to blood vessels, nerves.

▶ **Instruments.** Alternatives: plate, combined with a 2.7-mm lag screw; 2.7-mm cross screws. Locking plate system.

▶ **Position.** Supine. Foot in neutral position with toes pointing upward. A pelvic support and tilting the table can be used to achieve a better ankle position. Lower the contralateral foot. The foot lies with the edge of the heel over the end of the table.

Intraoperative radiographic imaging is only rarely needed.

▶ **Approach.** See ▶ Fig. 5.16.

▶ **Surgical technique.** See ▶ Fig. 5.17, ▶ Fig. 5.18, ▶ Fig. 5.19, ▶ Fig. 5.20, ▶ Fig. 5.21, ▶ Fig. 5.22, ▶ Fig. 5.23.

▶ **Postoperative aftercare.** A forefoot decompression shoe is used for 6 weeks. After that, radiographic imaging is performed for clearance to full weight bearing. Soft cushion insoles are used once foot swelling has subsided.

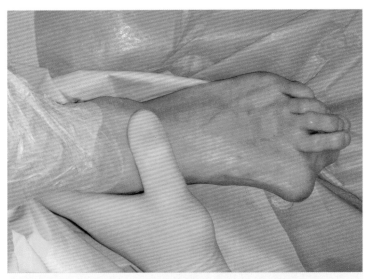

Fig. 5.15 Severe rheumatic splayfoot. Hallux valgus is no longer clinically correctable. Arthrodesis is indicated because of insufficient soft tissue.

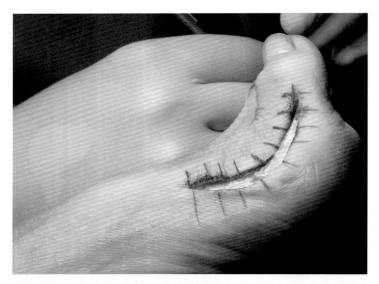

Fig. 5.16 A dorsomedial longitudinal skin incision is made starting ca. 3 cm proximal to the great toe proximal joint and continued distally over it. The dorsomedial neurovascular bundle is exposed. The sensory cutaneous nerve runs from dorsal to plantar, and crosses over the distal end of the more longitudinally oriented vessel.

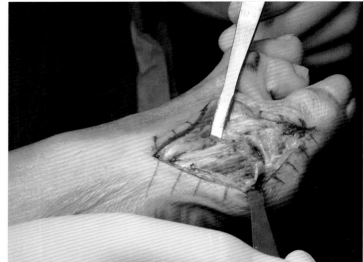

Fig. 5.17 The joint is exposed. Osteophytes are excised and, if necessary, a joint synovectomy is performed. The pseudoexostosis is resected tangential to the shaft axis. In contrast to a corrective osteotomy, the bony gutter is also resected here.

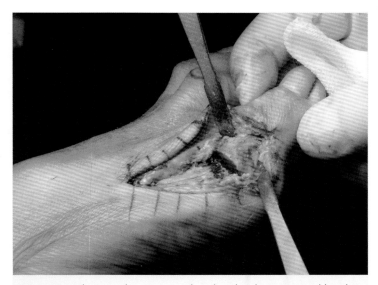

Fig. 5.18 Hohmann elevators are placed under the metatarsal head. A sparing osteotomy is performed on the joint surfaces. The shaft of the micro saw is used to guide the direction of the cut along the shaft axis, the blade being perpendicular to the saw. Depending upon the anatomical structure, the osteotomy is inclined approximately 3 to 4° relative to the shaft axis in order to achieve a distinct posterior extension of the toe. Follow the same procedure for the base of the proximal phalanx. If the joint still cannot be repositioned into a corrected position, additional soft tissue release must be performed. It is important to mobilize the sesamoid bone complex, since significant adhesions are usually present here. For severe secondary arthritic changes, we perform a reshaping arthroplasty.

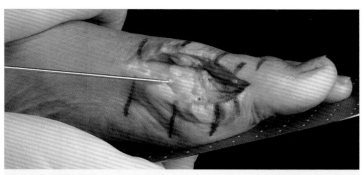

Fig. 5.19 The resultant correction is transfixed with a K-wire. The foot is placed on a flat surface, such as a surgical pan cover of approximately the same length, and alignment of the arthrodesis is confirmed in all planes. Repositioning of the foot is done under axial compression, in order to mimic the load during a footstep. The distance from the tip of the toe to the plate should be approximately 3 to 4 mm. The great toe should line up with the corrected remaining toes. The remaining mobility in the great toe distal joint is tested to ensure that it makes contact with the plate during plantar flexion and has at least 1 cm clearance from the plate during dorsiflexion.

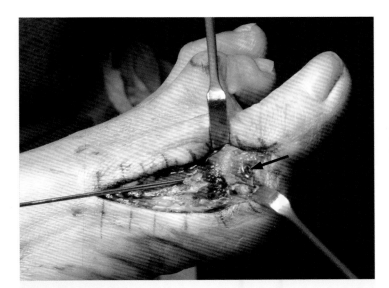

Fig. 5.20 The arthrodesis is adjusted and compressed. A 2.7-mm interfragmentary compression screw (arrow) is inserted from distal to proximal. This screw should be located in the plantar half of the shaft.

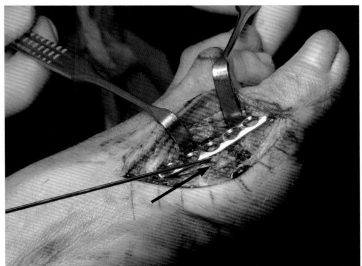

Fig. 5.21 A five-hole neutralization plate is attached. If the bones are severely osteoporotic, a locking plate can be attached on the dorsal side. An alternative technique is to place a second interfragmentary compression screw from proximal (arrow). We perform both techniques in combination if the bones are very osteoporotic.

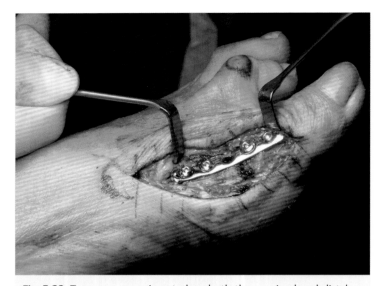

Fig. 5.22 Two screws are inserted on both the proximal and distal ends of the plate. Care must be taken with the second proximal screw, as it usually sits at the level of the sesamoid bone complex. For severely osteoporotic bone, the screw length must be measured carefully. If in doubt, it should be visually checked plantarly to avoid placement of an excessively long screw.

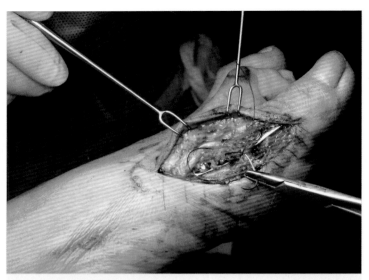

Fig. 5.23 A secure capsule closure is necessary for wound healing and to adequately cover the metal surfaces.

5.5 Great Toe Metatarsophalangeal Joint Prosthesis

▶ **Indication.** Larsen IV–V great toe proximal joint destruction with significant clinical symptoms. Hallux varus or valgus with severe rheumatic splayfoot.

▶ **Specific disclosures for patient consent.** Impaired wound healing. Prosthesis loosening. Infection with sequelae (necessitating prosthesis removal). Prosthesis breakage. Tendon injury. Injury to blood vessels and nerves.

▶ **Instruments.** Specific instruments according to the prosthesis system manufacturer.

▶ **Position.** Supine. Foot in neutral position with toes pointing upward. A pelvic support and tilting of the table can be used to achieve a better ankle position. Lower the contralateral foot. The foot is positioned with the edge of the heel over the end of the table.

Intraoperative radiologic imaging is only rarely needed.

▶ **Approach.** See ▶ Fig. 5.24.

▶ **Surgical technique.** See ▶ Fig. 5.25, ▶ Fig. 5.26, ▶ Fig. 5.27, ▶ Fig. 5.28, ▶ Fig. 5.29, ▶ Fig. 5.30, ▶ Fig. 5.31, ▶ Fig. 5.32, ▶ Fig. 5.33.

▶ **Postoperative aftercare.** A forefoot decompression shoe is used for 6 weeks. After that, radiologic imaging is performed for clearance to full weight bearing. Soft cushion insoles are used once foot swelling has subsided.

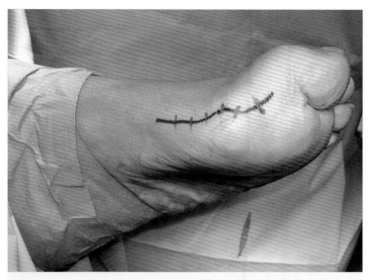

Fig. 5.24 A dorsomedial incision is made over the great toe proximal joint. The dorsomedial neurovascular bundle is exposed. In particular, the cutaneous nerve is exposed and retracted off to the side (see also Chapter 5.2).

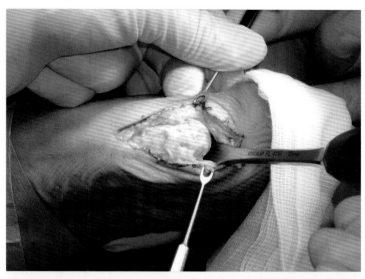

Fig. 5.25 Longitudinal capsulotomy and proximal joint exposure. A proximal joint arthrolysis is performed first. Contractures are released, particularly from the lateral side.

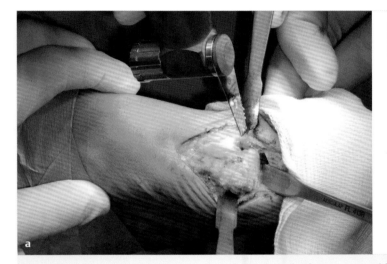

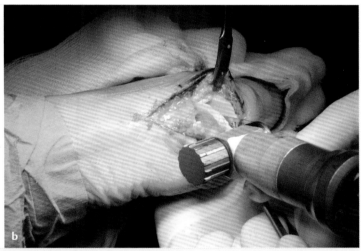

Fig. 5.26 (a,b) A sparing osteotomy is performed on the first metatarsal head and the base of the proximal joint **(b)**.

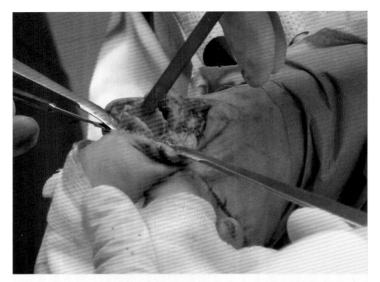

Fig. 5.27 A sparing osteotomy is performed on the base of the first proximal joint.

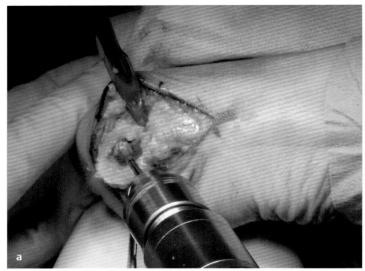

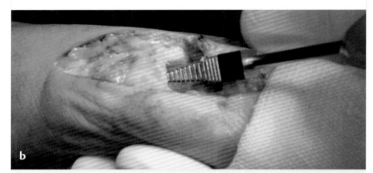

Fig. 5.28 (a,b) The proximal segment is reamed open using the appropriate reamer, or a bur if needed.

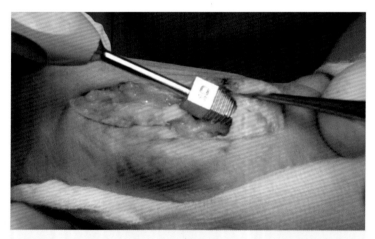

Fig. 5.29 The distal segment is reamed open using the corresponding reamer.

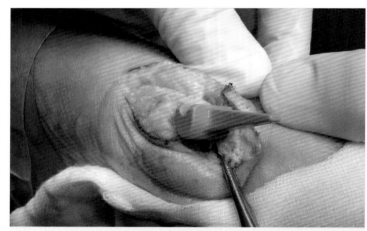

Fig. 5.30 The trial implants are inserted. The position and tension of the implant are checked as well as mobility and the ability to bear load.

5

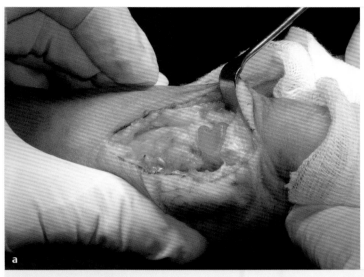
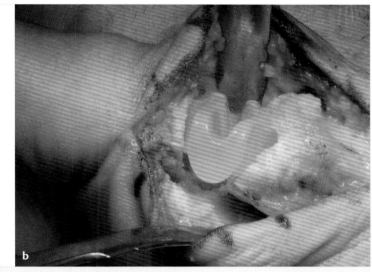

Fig. 5.31 (a,b) Implantation of the prosthesis. The stability is checked.

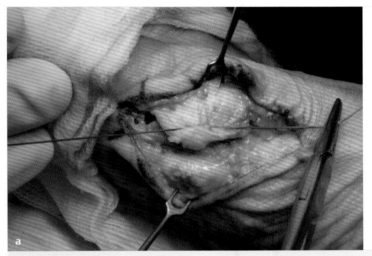
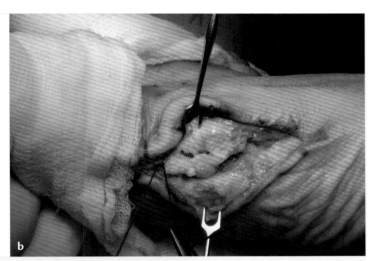

Fig. 5.32 (a,b) The capsule is meticulously closed (risk of dislocation). The sesamoid bone complex is repositioned with a cerclage fibreux procedure.

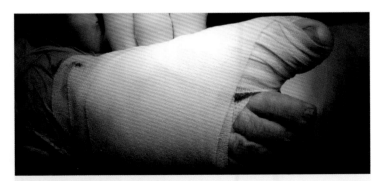

Fig. 5.33 Splint bandage dressing.

5.6 Helal Osteotomy

▶ **Indication.** Severe therapy-resistant metatarsalgia. No severe Larsen IV–V destruction of the metatarsal heads.

▶ **Specific disclosures for patient consent.** Impaired wound healing. Pseudarthroses. Infection. Tendon injury. Injury to blood vessels and nerves. Recurrence of metatarsalgia. Head necrosis.

▶ **Position.** Supine. Foot in neutral position with toes pointing upward. A pelvic support and tilting of the table can be used to achieve a better ankle position. Lower the contralateral foot. The foot is positioned with the edge of the heel over the end of the table.

▶ **Approach.** See ▶ Fig. 5.34.

▶ **Surgical technique.** See ▶ Fig. 5.35, ▶ Fig. 5.36.

▶ **Postoperative aftercare.** As much weight bearing as the pain allows. Soft cushion insoles are used once foot swelling has subsided.

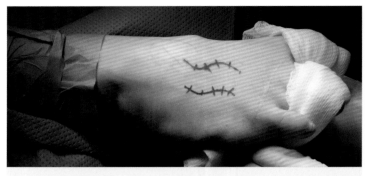

Fig. 5.34 Two S-shaped curved incisions are made over the base of the metatarsal, usually between the second and third and the third and fourth metatarsals.

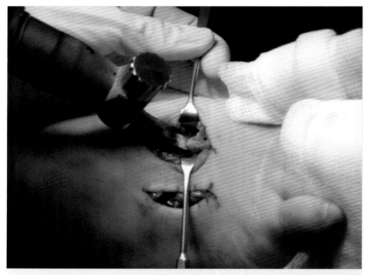

Fig. 5.35 The base of the second metatarsal is exposed from proximal to the middle third. The extensor tendon is held to the side. The saw is positioned, and the osteotomy is performed from proximal to distal at an angle of approximately 45°. Osteosynthesis is not performed in the Helal procedure; the head is repositioned using pressure.

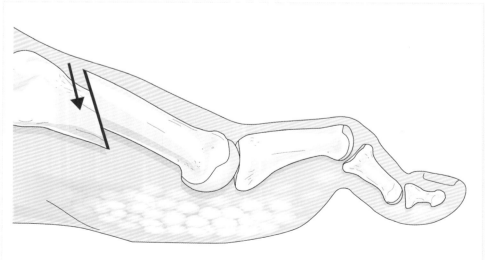

Fig. 5.36 Schematic drawing of the Helal osteotomy. The arrow indicates the direction of displacement of the osteotomy.

5.7 Weil Osteotomy

▶ **Indication.** Severe rheumatic splayfoot. Pronounced metatarsalgias. Metatarsophalangeal (MTP) joint dislocation. Soft tissues must be correctable. Larsen I–II (III) destruction.

▶ **Specific disclosures for patient consent.** Impaired wound healing. Pseudarthrosis. Metatarsal head necrosis with sequelae. Recurrence. Joint stiffness. Tendon incompetence. Infection. Tendon injury. Injury to blood vessels and nerves.

▶ **Instruments.** Screw 2.0-mm with flat-head or specialized countersinkable headless screws equipped with two different threads ("Herbert" screw).

▶ **Position.** Supine, foot in neutral position with toes pointing upward. A pelvic support and tilting of the table can be used to achieve a better ankle position. Lower the contralateral foot. The foot is positioned with the edge of the heel over the end of the table.

Intraoperative radiologic imaging is only rarely needed.

▶ **Approach.** See ▶ Fig. 5.37, ▶ Fig. 5.38.

▶ **Surgical technique.** See ▶ Fig. 5.39, ▶ Fig. 5.40, ▶ Fig. 5.41, ▶ Fig. 5.42, ▶ Fig. 5.44, ▶ Fig. 5.45.

▶ **Postoperative aftercare.** Immediate mobilization exercises are important postoperatively to prevent joint stiffness. An orthotic to protect the soft tissues is worn full-time for 6 weeks, and then at nighttime only for an additional 6 weeks. Forefoot decompression shoe is used for 6 weeks. Then, radiologic imaging is done for clearance to full weight bearing. Soft cushion insoles are used once foot swelling has subsided. See also ▶ Fig. 5.43.

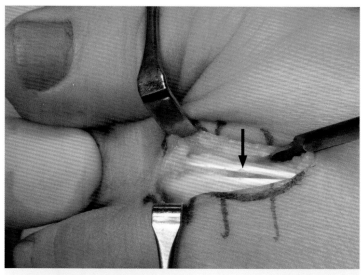

Fig. 5.37 The second toe is usually accessed via the **S**-shaped incision used for a first toe adductor tenotomy. Otherwise, an intermetatarsal skin incision between the third and fourth toes can be used as a surgical approach to the other toes. An alternative is a fully transverse incision to access all of the proximal joints (see also Chapter 5.8.1, dorsal approach, metatarsal head resection). Postoperative immobilization is in a prefabricated plaster alignment splint. The extensor tendon (arrow) is split longitudinally. This tendon is easier to reconstruct than the more vulnerable retinaculum when closing inflamed rheumatoid tissue. For lateral displacement of the extensor apparatus (usually fibular), the extensor tendon is entered on the fibular side. Duplication of the tibial section is attempted during closure.

5

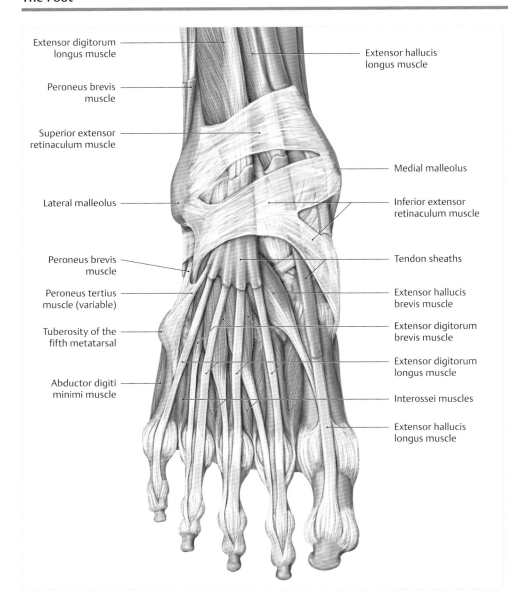

Extensor digitorum longus muscle

Extensor hallucis longus muscle

Peroneus brevis muscle

Superior extensor retinaculum muscle

Medial malleolus

Lateral malleolus

Inferior extensor retinaculum muscle

Peroneus brevis muscle

Tendon sheaths

Peroneus tertius muscle (variable)

Extensor hallucis brevis muscle

Tuberosity of the fifth metatarsal

Extensor digitorum brevis muscle

Extensor digitorum longus muscle

Abductor digiti minimi muscle

Interossei muscles

Extensor hallucis longus muscle

Fig. 5.38 Anatomy of the extensor tendons. A Z-shaped tenotomy is performed on the extensor digitorum longus. If necessary, the extensor digitorum brevis muscle can be tenotomized and then sutured together with the extensor digitorum longus muscle in a tension-free manner. (From: Schünke M, Schulte E, Schumacher U. Prometheus. LernAtlas der Anatomie: Allgemeine Anatomie und Bewegungssysteme. Illustrated by M. Voll and K. Wesker. 2nd edition. Stuttgart: Thieme; 2007.)

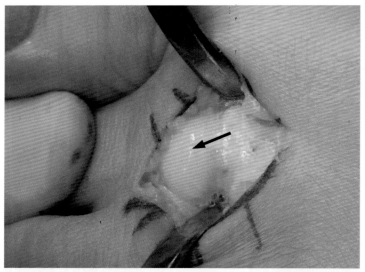

Fig. 5.39 A longitudinal capsulotomy of the metatarsophalangeal joint is performed. Synovectomy of the joint is carried out if needed. Extensive arthrolysis of the joint is seen here. If the joint is not reducible, the dorsal section of the ligament apparatus may need to be released. Hohmann elevators are placed under the metatarsal head (arrow) in order to avoid injuring the neighboring structures during osteotomy.

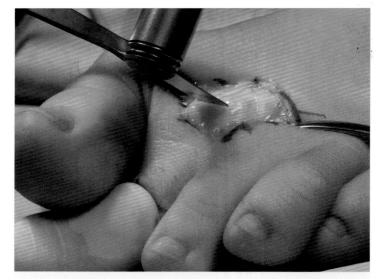

Fig. 5.40 The osteotomy is preferably performed tangential to the shaft axis. Caveat: too steep an incline of the osteotomy leads to plantarization of the metatarsal head and increased metatarsalgia. In order to counteract plantarization, the osteotomy is performed with a double-thickness saw blade or a second parallel osteotomy that removes an additional 2-mm segment.

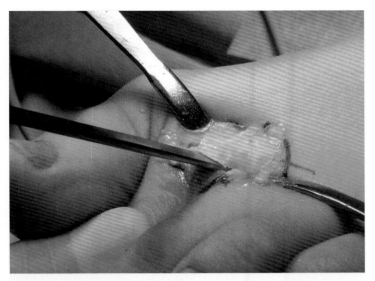

Fig. 5.41 The osteotomies are carefully mobilized using a chisel. No high forces should be applied on the dorsal side as these jeopardize the thinner dorsal fragment.

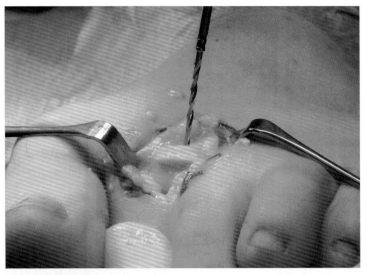

Fig. 5.42 Hohmann elevators are not used during repositioning since they impede physiologic repositioning maneuvers. The amount of proximal displacement is determined from the preoperative radiograph. The goal is to achieve a physiologic overall alignment of all of the metatarsal heads. The necessary distance in millimeters can be calculated preoperatively from the radiograph and then translated in situ. The fragments have a tendency to move spontaneously into the desired position if they have been properly released. A lateral displacement of the head can be accommodated with this technique. Here the metatarsal head is displaced laterally, slightly in the direction of the luxated side and can thus better offset the dislocation.

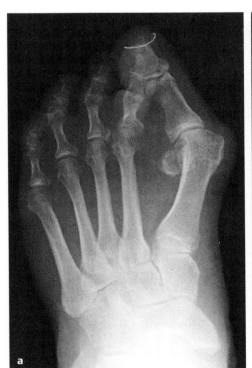
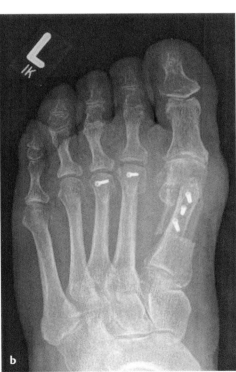

Fig. 5.43 Radiographs. **(a)** Preoperative. **(b)** Postoperative.

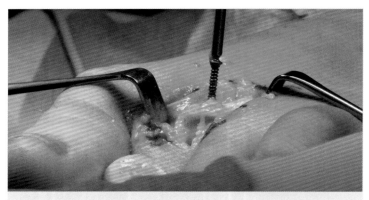

Fig. 5.44 As a rule, the surgeon can easily fixate the reduction by simultaneously flexing the affected toe with the other hand and pressing from plantar toward dorsal against the easily palpable metatarsal head. The osteotomy fragments are fixed with a 2.0-mm screw. The typical screw length is 12 mm for the second–fourth toes, and 10 mm for the fifth toe. The screws should be set up prior to drilling so that they can be fixed immediately after drilling. This prevents the reduction from slipping. The soft rheumatoid bone does not tolerate multiple drillings.

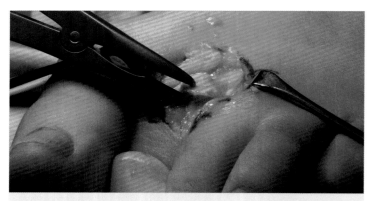

Fig. 5.45 The bony protrusions are removed. The excess bone is removed, and the resultant metatarsal length can be compared with the amount of shortening required based on preoperative radiologic imaging. The extensor tendon is sutured.

5.8 Resection of Metatarsal Heads II–V

Metatarsal head resection via the plantar or dorsal operative approach produces excellent results. The choice of approach depends primarily on the experience of the surgeon with the respective procedure.

5.8.1 Dorsal Approach (Hoffman)

▶ **Indication.** Larsen III–V destruction with significant clinical symptoms; severe rheumatic splayfoot.

▶ **Specific disclosures for patient consent.** Impaired wound healing. Infection. Tendon injury. Injury to blood vessels, nerves. Recurrence. Neocallus formation.

▶ **Instruments.** Fixation with a 1.4-mm K-wire for severe contractures.

▶ **Position.** Supine. Foot in neutral position with toes pointing upward. A pelvic support and tilting of the table can be used to achieve a better ankle position. Lower the contralateral foot. The foot is positioned with the edge of the heel over the end of the table.

▶ **Approach.** See ▶ Fig. 5.46.

▶ **Surgical technique.** See ▶ Fig. 5.47, ▶ Fig. 5.48, ▶ Fig. 5.49, ▶ Fig. 5.50, ▶ Fig. 5.51, ▶ Fig. 5.52.

▶ **Postoperative aftercare.** A plaster positioning splint with foot in dorsiflexion is used to avoid placing pressure on the incision during the wound healing phase. A forefoot decompression shoe is used for 6 weeks. Soft cushion insoles are used once foot swelling has subsided.

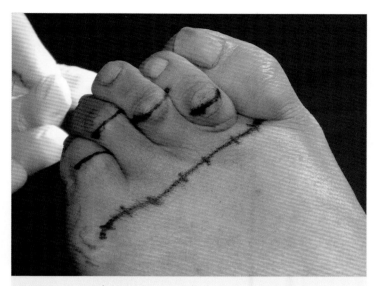

Fig. 5.46 Surgical incisions are marked. A transverse incision is planned for the metatarsal heads. Another option is two longitudinal incisions in the second–third and fourth–fifth intermetatarsal spaces.

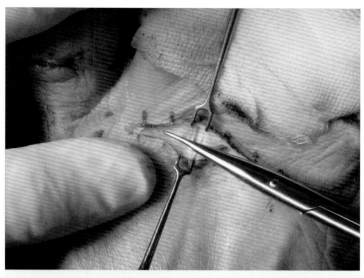

Fig. 5.47 Exposure of the extensor tendon. A Z-shaped tenotomy and elongation are typically performed. The metatarsophalangeal joints are usually displaced. The proximal phalanx is then easily palpable. The joint capsule is divided transversely. Using manual longitudinal traction on the toes, extensive arthrolysis is performed on the joint until it can be repositioned. The collateral ligaments may also need to be divided. If one encounters difficulty, a periosteal elevator can be inserted in the joint space and used as a lever to perform the reduction.

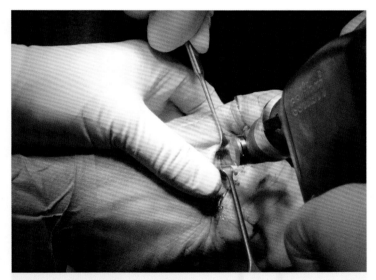

Fig. 5.48 Metatarsal head osteotomy. The osteotomy plane is inclined from dorsal distally toward plantar proximally.

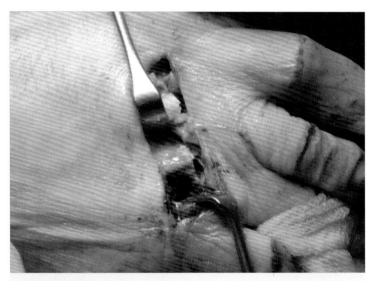

Fig. 5.49 After resection of the metatarsal head, the soft tissue release is completed: capsule mobilization is continued until the toes spontaneously move into position.

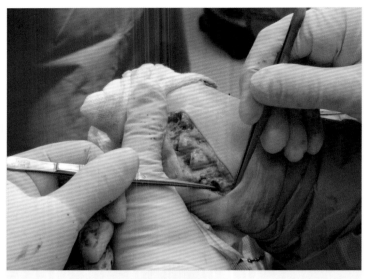

Fig. 5.50 Mobilization of the plantar capsule usually takes place after resection of the metatarsal head. To prevent the formation of sharp edges, the metatarsal head is resected in the same manner as in the plantar approach, from dorsal distally toward plantar proximally, at a 30° incline. A vertical osteotomy is frequently performed on the fifth metatarsal head to avoid leaving any sharp points.

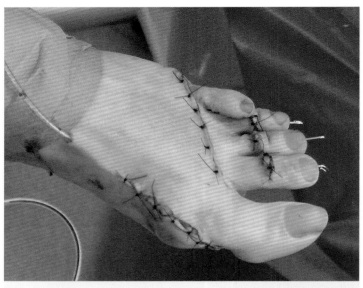

Fig. 5.51 A Swanson prosthesis was implanted in the first toe. As a rule, only the proximal interphalangeal (PIP) joint arthrodesis is stabilized with a K-wire. In this case, the second to fourth toes are fixed with a K-wire due to severe contracture. The fifth toe must also be secured with a K-wire, since it will not spontaneously move into the correct position.

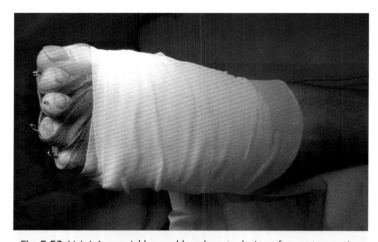

Fig. 5.52 Vainio's special layered bandage technique for postoperative stabilization of the toes. The pull of the bandage slings imparts traction toward the great toe in the plantar direction.

5.8.2 Plantar Approach (Tillman)

▶ **Indication.** Larsen III–V destruction with significant clinical symptoms. Severe metatarsalgias. Severe rheumatic splayfoot.

▶ **Specific disclosures for patient consent.** Impaired wound healing. Infection. Tendon injury. Injury to blood vessels, nerves. Recurrence. Neocallus formation.

▶ **Instruments.** Fixation with a 1.4-mm K-wire for severe contractures.

▶ **Position.** Supine. Foot in neutral position with toes pointing upward. A pelvic support and tilting of the table can be used to achieve a better ankle position. Lower the contralateral foot. The foot lies with the edge of the heel over the end of the table.

▶ **Approach.** See ▶ Fig. 5.53.

▶ **Surgical technique.** See ▶ Fig. 5.54, ▶ Fig. 5.55, ▶ Fig. 5.56, ▶ Fig. 5.57, ▶ Fig. 5.58, ▶ Fig. 5.59, ▶ Fig. 5.60, ▶ Fig. 5.61.

▶ **Postoperative aftercare.** A forefoot decompression shoe is used for 6 weeks. Soft cushion insoles are used once foot swelling has subsided.

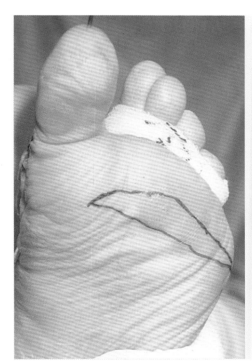

Fig. 5.53 An oval-shaped incision is made directly over the thick corns on the sole of the foot. The size of the skin to be excised from the affected area is matched to the extent of proximal phalanx displacement. For pronounced skin changes, this type of incision provides an additional dermodesis effect.

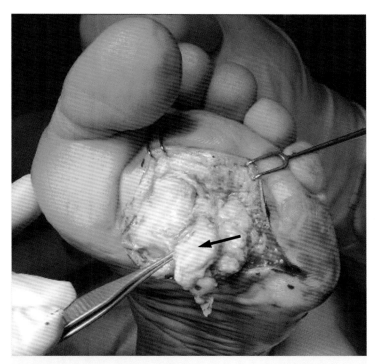

Fig. 5.54 Enormous bursae frequently arise directly under the metatarsal heads (arrow). These are carefully extirpated. The remaining plantar fatty tissue should be completely preserved during the resection. With pronounced rheumatoid splayfoot, the tendons and neurovascular bundle are usually displaced interdigitally.

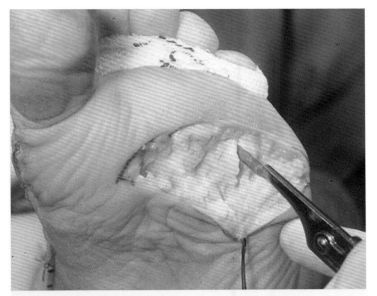

Fig. 5.55 The joint capsule is exposed along with the flexor tendon apparatus. A longitudinal incision is made. With a severe deformity, the flexor tendons are displaced between the metatarsal heads. The less pronounced the rheumatoid changes, the more likely the tendons are to remain in their original position. The tendons are exposed and held off to the side.

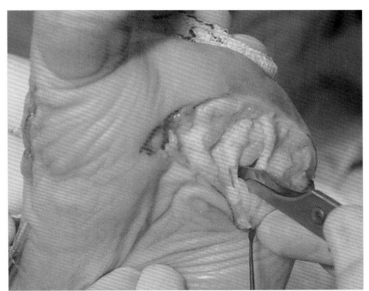

Fig. 5.56 The proximal adhesions of the joint capsule are released with a no. 11 blade. This should be done under direct vision, particularly for severe contractures. Otherwise, the laterally displaced flexor tendons are put at risk.

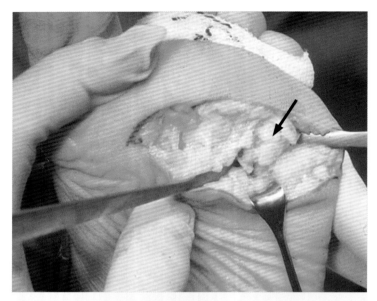

Fig. 5.57 Two Hohmann elevators are placed on the bone directly under the metatarsal heads. The arrow shows the metatarsal head with inflammatory changes. Caveat: the dislocated tendons must be securely held to the side and protected. Hohmann elevators are positioned at the level of the osteotomy.

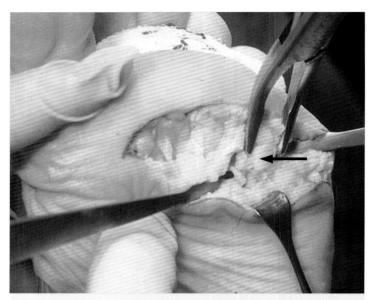

Fig. 5.58 The plantar projection of the metatarsal head (arrow) is removed with a Luer. In this way the metatarsal head to metatarsal shaft transition can be accurately exposed; otherwise, plantar projection is larger than the head–shaft transition and too much bone is often resected with the first osteotomy.

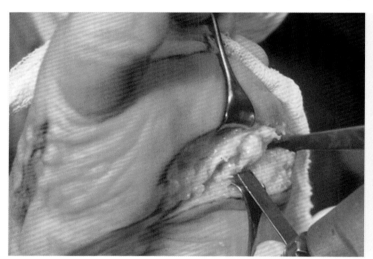

Fig. 5.59 An osteotomy of the metatarsal head is performed exactly at the shaft transition point. The osteotomy is performed with an upward incline from plantar proximal toward dorsal distal. Sharp edges must be smoothed with the Luer. There must be enough room to reduce the displaced proximal phalanxes without tension. Otherwise, the capsule must be completely mobilized dorsally or further resected. A vertical osteotomy is usually performed on the fifth metatarsal head in order to avoid creating any sharp edges. A sharp release is performed to free the resected metatarsal head as much as possible. A towel clamp is used to hold the head because the Luer usually destroys osteoporotic bone. The head is extracted from the surrounding capsule tissue in a stepwise fashion. Removal of smaller osteoporotic fragments is considerably more difficult if the head cannot be removed in one piece.

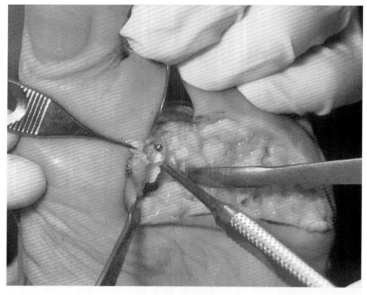

Fig. 5.60 Reconstruction of the soft tissues. The dislocated tendon is recentered. The capsule is plicated with an intersecting x-suture in order to achieve a better soft tissue correction of the neoarthrosis.

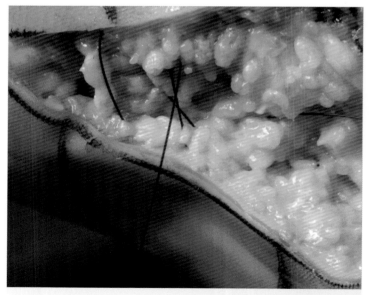

Fig. 5.61 Reconstruction of the plantar fat pad is particularly important. This is mobilized so as to relocate it over the resected head and allow for a successful procedure. The technique usually involves an interrupted x-suture. The skin is sewn together with a sturdy suture (3–0); thin sutures erode during mobilization.

5.9 Great Toe Interphalangeal Joint Arthrodesis

▶ **Indication.** Rheumatoid hallux valgus interphalangeus deformity. Larsen III–V destruction with significant clinical symptoms. See also ▶ Fig. 5.62, ▶ Fig. 5.63.

▶ **Specific disclosures for patient consent.** Impaired wound healing. Pseudarthrosis. Infection. Tendon injury. Injury to blood vessels and nerves.

▶ **Instruments.** Fixation with a 3.5-mm or 4.5-mm cancellous screw.

▶ **Position.** Supine. Foot in neutral position with toes pointing upward. A pelvic support and tilting of the table can be used to achieve a better ankle position. Lower the contralateral foot. The foot is positioned with the edge of the heel over the end of the table.

▶ **Approach.** See ▶ Fig. 5.64.

▶ **Surgical technique.** See ▶ Fig. 5.65, ▶ Fig. 5.66, ▶ Fig. 5.67, ▶ Fig. 5.68.

▶ **Postoperative aftercare.** A forefoot decompression shoe is used for 6 weeks. Soft cushion insoles are used once foot swelling has subsided.

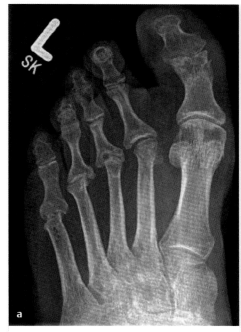
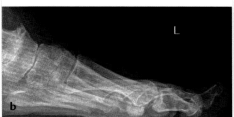

Fig. 5.62 (a,b) Pronounced rheumatoid forefoot deformity. The splayfoot with destroyed metatarsal heads is clinically asymptomatic. The main etiology is a combination of hallux valgus interphalangeus deformity along with interphalangeal (IP) joint destruction.

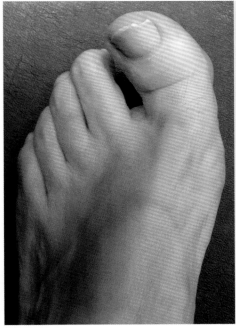

Fig. 5.63 Clinical picture.

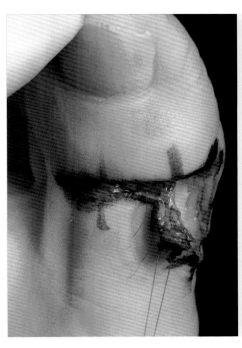

Fig. 5.64 An L-shaped skin incision is made and the wound edges are reinforced with stay-sutures A Y-shaped incision is also possible.

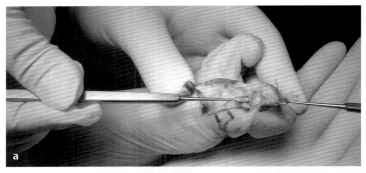
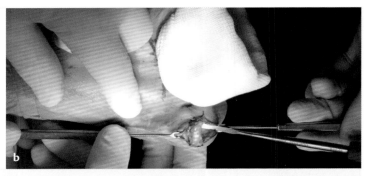

Fig. 5.65 Transverse capsulotomy. If necessary, a synovectomy of the joint is performed. The joint surfaces are exposed and scored, and the ligament apparatus can be detached if necessary. The cartilage is removed from the joint surfaces with a Luer. Once the joint surfaces have been decorticated, they are reduced into a corrected position. The arthrodesis configuration is verified clinically.

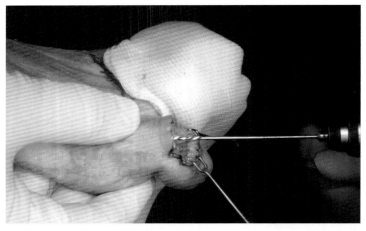
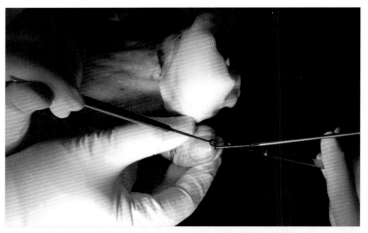

Fig. 5.66 A 2.7 to 3.5-mm drill is used to drill through the center of the distal fragment from proximal to distal. This is accomplished via a stab incision approximately 1 mm plantar to the nail. The drill is then redirected through the drill hole and positioned in the middle of the proximal phalanx under direct vision. The proximal phalanx is then drilled down its center. Care must be taken with rheumatoid bones.

Fig. 5.67 The same procedure is performed with the 3.5 to 4.5-mm cancellous screw: Following insertion through the distal phalanx, it is brought into the central drill hole of the proximal phalanx. This is necessary because, without pilot holes, new canals can also easily be created in rheumatoid bone.

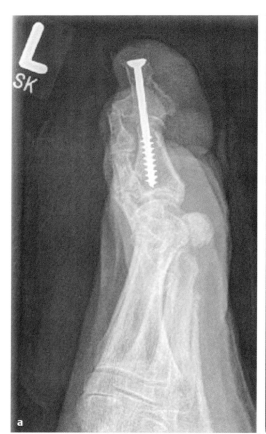
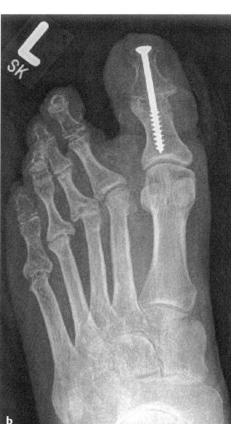

Fig. 5.68 (a,b) The screws must be of sufficient length. In our experience, the risk of pseudarthrosis is significantly increased if the screws are too short.

5.10 Proximal Interphalangeal Joint Arthrodesis

▶ **Indication.** Rheumatic claw toe deformity (▶ Fig. 5.69).

▶ **Specific disclosures for patient consent.** Impaired wound healing. Infection.

We usually perform an arthrodesis. The Hohmann osteotomy technique leads to a higher recurrence rate in rheumatoid patients who have very contracted structures.

▶ **Instruments.** Fixation with a double-pointed 1.2-mm K-wire.

▶ **Position.** Supine. Foot in neutral position with toes pointing upward. A pelvic support and tilting of the table can be used to achieve a better ankle position. Lower the contralateral foot. The foot is positioned with the edge of the heel over the end of the table.

▶ **Surgical technique.** See ▶ Fig. 5.70, ▶ Fig. 5.71, ▶ Fig. 5.72, ▶ Fig. 5.73, ▶ Fig. 5.74.

▶ **Postoperative aftercare.** K-wire is left in place for 6 weeks; a shoe splint for 6 weeks. Soft cushion insoles are used once foot swelling has subsided.

5

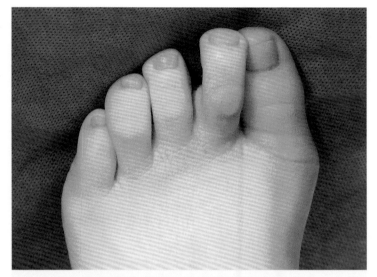

Fig. 5.69 Clinically apparent thick corn formation on the proximal second interphalangeal joint.

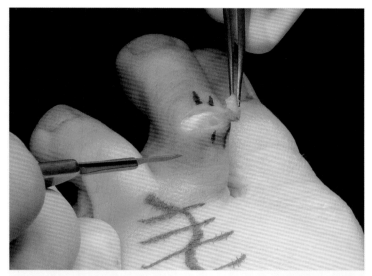

Fig. 5.70 An oval-shaped transverse incision is made over the corn to excise the affected area. A longitudinal skin incision is also an option. This type of incision is frequently made tangential to the incision used for revision of the proximal joint. Drawn here is an **S**-shaped approach to the second and third proximal joints.

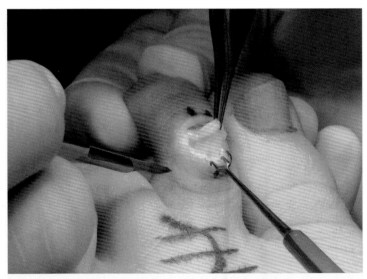

Fig. 5.71 The extensor tendon is divided horizontally.

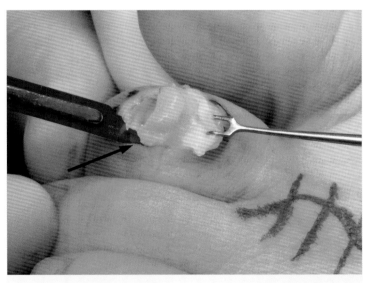

Fig. 5.72 The ligament apparatus (arrow) of the joint is released medially and laterally.

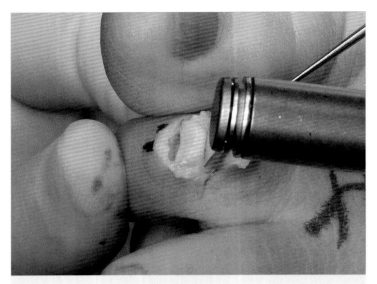

Fig. 5.73 The proximal joint segment is resected with the saw perpendicular to the shaft axis. Liston scissors are more likely to crush the rheumatoid bone.

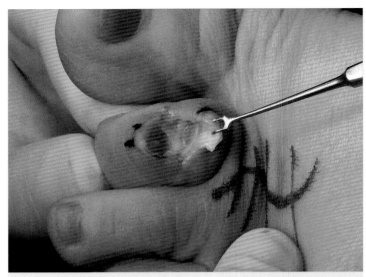

Fig. 5.74 Cartilage is removed from the distal joint segment down to cancellous bone. The double-tipped K-wire is first drilled through the distal phalanx from proximally. It is then gripped by the drill and fixed into the middle phalanx under direct vision. If we opt for an osteoclasis instead of an arthrodesis, this position correction is also fixated with a percutaneously introduced interosseous wire. The extensor tendon is sutured. The skin is sutured to create a dermodesis effect.

Chapter 6

The Ankle

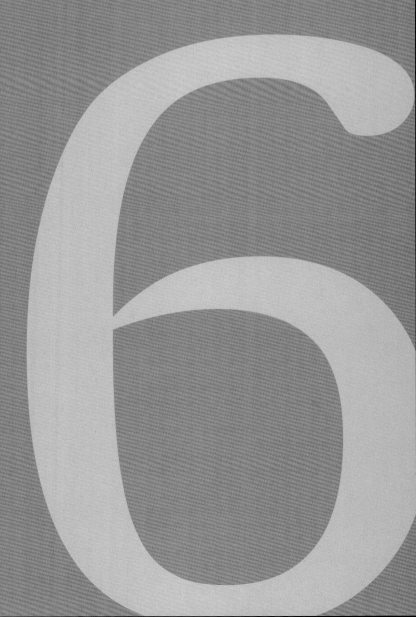

6 The Ankle

S. Sell, S. Rehart, A. Lehr, V. Crnic

6.1 Arthroscopic and Open Synovectomy/Tenosynovectomy of the Tibiotalar Joint

▶ **Indication.** Synovitis of the tibiotalar joint and/or tenosynovitis with maximum Larsen Stage II destruction. Patients frequently do not have any subjective clinical symptoms.

Detection of isolated synovitis of the tibiotalar joint is often very difficult clinically, and frequently requires additional diagnostic investigation such as ultrasonography and MRI. Isolated synovitis of the tibiotalar joint can usually be addressed arthroscopically.

▶ **Specific disclosures for patient consent.** Tendon injury or rupture (also secondary). Blood vessel, nerve injury. Recurrent synovitis.

Open synovectomy is almost always performed if the synovitis is accompanied by tenosynovitis.

The patient must be informed of the potential for intraoperative conversion to an open procedure.

▶ **Position.** Supine. Ankle in neutral position with toes pointed toward the ceiling. It is usually necessary to place a positioning roll under the ipsilateral buttock in order to compensate for external rotation of hip. A contralateral pelvic support and tilting of the table can be used to achieve a better ankle position. The ankle joint rests approximately 3 to 5 cm over the end of the table.

▶ **Approach.** For arthroscopic synovectomy, see ▶ Fig. 6.1, ▶ Fig. 6.2. For open synovectomy, see ▶ Fig. 6.8, ▶ Fig. 6.9, ▶ Fig. 6.10.

▶ **Surgical technique.** For arthroscopic synovectomy, see ▶ Fig. 6.3, ▶ Fig. 6.4, ▶ Fig. 6.5, ▶ Fig. 6.6, ▶ Fig. 6.7. For open synovectomy, see ▶ Fig. 6.11.

▶ **Postoperative aftercare.** Mobilize under partial load for 3 weeks to allow for synovial regeneration. Radiosynoviorthesis is usually recommended 6 weeks after arthroscopic synovectomy.

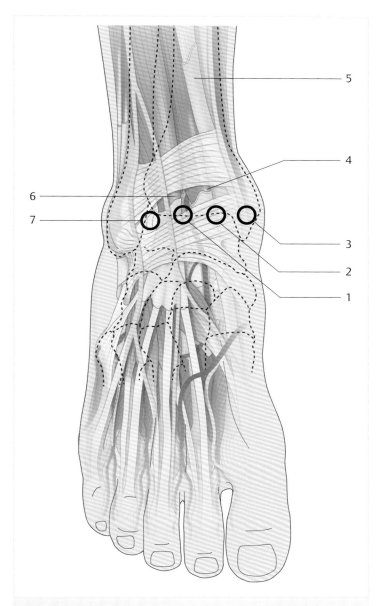

Fig. 6.1 An anterolateral port is usually placed first after a stab incision. Next, an anteromedial port is placed under direct vision. The joint can be insufflated with normal saline first if the joint is difficult to localize. Distraction mechanisms are often unnecessary. Posterior approaches are generally avoided, unless the preoperative MRI scan demonstrates pronounced dorsal synovitis. The instruments usually need to be switched several times between the portals in order to perform a thorough synovectomy. 1, Anterocentral portal. 2, Accessory anterior portal. 3, Anteromedial portal. 4, Extensor hallucis longus tendon. 5, Anterior tibial tendon. 6, Extensor digitorum longus tendon. 7, Anterolateral portal.

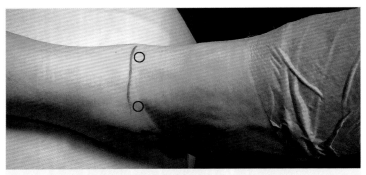

Fig. 6.2 Anteromedial portal (medial to the anterior tibial tendon). Anterolateral portal (lateral to the extensor digitorum longus tendon). If needed, the joint is first insufflated with normal saline using an injection needle.

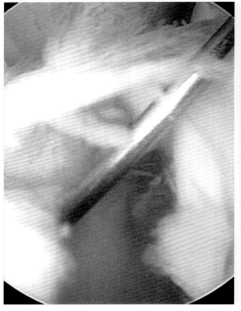

Fig. 6.3 After placement of the lateral portal, the medial portal is placed under direct vision. This is frequently more difficult due to extensive synovitis.

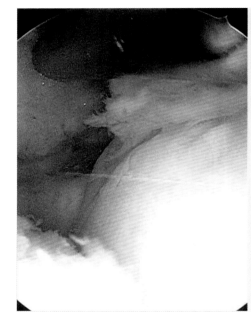

Fig. 6.4 The entire ankle joint is examined. Synovectomy is first performed in the central portion of the joint, along the tibial crest and talus. This frequently results in a substantial improvement in visibility.

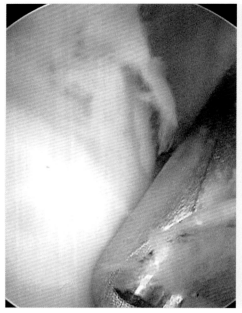

Fig. 6.5 The synovectomy is completed in the medial and lateral compartment.

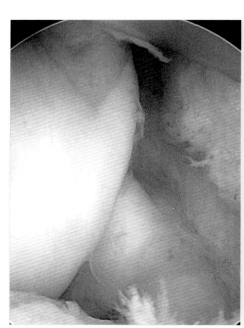

Fig. 6.6 Completed synovectomy. The cartilage is still in relatively good condition.

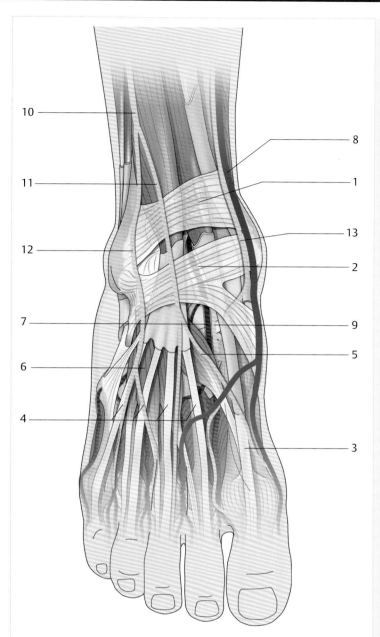

Fig. 6.7 Schematic drawing of the anatomy. It is important to pay attention to the exact location of the vessel and nerve structures when planning the anatomical approaches.
1, Superior extensor retinaculum. 2, Inferior extensor retinaculum. 3, Extensor hallucis longus muscle tendon. 4, Extensor digitorum longus muscle tendon. 5, Extensor hallucis brevis muscle. 6, Extensor digitorum brevis muscle. 7, Dorsalis pedis artery. 8, Greater saphenous vein. 9, Deep peroneal nerve. 10, Superficial peroneal nerve. 11, Intermediate dorsal cutaneous nerve. 12, Medial dorsal cutaneous nerve. 13, Saphenous nerve.

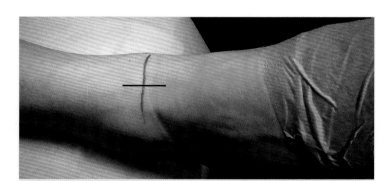

Fig. 6.8 Following palpation, a midline incision is made at the level of the anterior tibial muscle tendon. The position of the tibiotalar joint is determined by palpation during movement, and then marked.

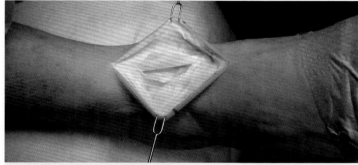

Fig. 6.9 Flexor retinaculum. Anterior tibial muscle tendon. Dissection of the subcutaneous tissue must be undertaken carefully because the superficial peroneal nerve runs extrafascially from proximal lateral to medial distal. If there are significant inflammatory changes and major displacement, it is advisable to deliberately expose the nerve and hold it to the side. Otherwise, the nerve is vulnerable in the distal area of the incision. The extensor retinaculum is exposed and divided at the level of the anterior tibial muscle. The tibia is accessed behind the anterior tibial muscle tendon. Dissection is started as far proximal as possible, because the distance to the neurovascular bundle is greater there. Dissection is then continued distally. This allows the neurovascular bundle to be retracted laterally (see ► Fig. 6.7). Often a synovectomy is required because the tendons are severely altered from synovitis.

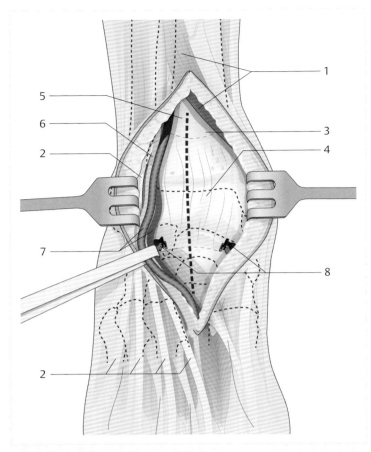

Fig. 6.10 Schematic drawing of the approach. 1, Extensor hallucis longus muscle. 2, Extensor digitorum longus muscle tendon. 3, Crural fascia. 4, Talocrural joint capsule. 5, Tibia. 6, Deep peroneal nerve. 7, Anterior tibial artery and vein. 8, Anterior medial malleolar and lateral malleolar artery and vein.

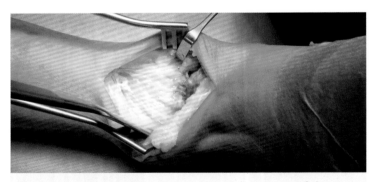

Fig. 6.11 It is important to ensure adequate hemostasis of the numerous vessels that cross in front of the joint when it is opened. Severe synovitis frequently leads to an increased number of blood vessels. The surgical site is then held open with a large spreader. Caveat: keep retractor tension to a minimum to avoid impaired wound healing. Synovectomy is performed under distraction to allow access to all of the compartments of the rheumatic joint, particularly the posteromedial areas and the lateral compartment. The joint structures are frequently elongated due to inflammation.

6.2 Tibiotalar Joint Prosthesis

▶ **Indication.** Larsen III–V destruction with significant clinical symptoms. Less than 15° axial deformity if possible. Severe deformities frequently require additional procedures, such as a simultaneous correction arthrodesis of the subtalar joint.

▶ **Specific disclosures for patient consent.** Prosthetic loosening. Tendon rupture (also secondary). Dislocation of the liner. Medial, lateral malleolar fractures (particular risk in rheumatic patients). Infection with sequelae. Blood vessel and nerve injury.

▶ **Instruments.** Prosthesis system from the manufacturer of choice. A TARIC prosthesis manufactured by Implantcast is shown here.

▶ **Position.** Supine. Ankle in neutral position with toes pointed toward the ceiling. It is usually necessary to place a positioning roll under the ipsilateral buttock in order to compensate for external rotation of hip. A radiograph may be needed.

▶ **Surgical techniques.** See ▶ Fig. 6.12, ▶ Fig. 6.13, ▶ Fig. 6.14, ▶ Fig. 6.15, ▶ Fig. 6.16, ▶ Fig. 6.17, ▶ Fig. 6.18, ▶ Fig. 6.19.

▶ **Approach for ligament instability.** Joint dislocations are rarely due to supramalleolar causes in rheumatoid patients.

Any axial deviation or deformity of the subtalar joint must be corrected prior to balancing the talotibial joint. If the subtalar joint is intact, correction may involve a calcaneal osteotomy. Should the destruction also involve the subtalar joint, arthrodesis with correction of the axis is recommended (see Chapter 6.4). This can be performed as a one-stage or two-stage procedure.

Once these causes are ruled out, correction can typically be performed articularly.

The largest portion of the misalignment is corrected and aligned as follows:
- Removal of all osteophytes.
- Release of all soft tissue adhesions (extensive arthrolysis).
- Bone resection with the ankle in neutral position, which may allow for partial correction of the resected bone.

▶ **Valgus.** Valgus deformity is more frequent in rheumatic patients. The correction is similar to that for a knee prosthesis.
- Deformity is caused by a bony defect and the medial ligament is still intact: further intervention is usually not necessary. If there are indications of lateral ligament instability, it may be necessary to perform a plication of the ligament structures or a ligament repair.
- Medial ligament insufficiency: a medial ligament plication or augmentation is performed, depending upon the severity. Endoprosthetic replacement of the tibiotalar joint is not an option if there is severe instability of the medial ligament.

▶ **Varus.** Varus deformities are relatively uncommon in rheumatic patients. Persistent instability following a standard approach is usually due to a deltoid ligament contracture. Medial malleolar corrective elongation osteotomy and realignment via an elevated liner are worth considering.

▶ **Postoperative aftercare.** Immediate full-range mobilization. For a stable endoprosthesis, mobilization with full weight bearing in a stability shoe (VACOped, for example) for 6 weeks. Another option is mobilization in a walking cast boot.

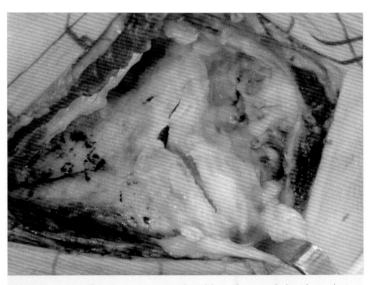

Fig. 6.12 A midline incision is made, although a medial or lateral approach is also possible. For description of the approach, see Chapter 6.1. Removal of all osteophytes is done first so as to obtain a good overview of the joint. It is important to release all of the adhesions. A large portion of the misalignment can be corrected by osteophyte removal and soft tissue release.

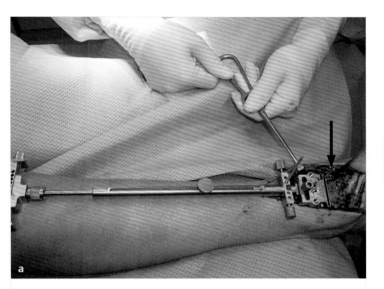

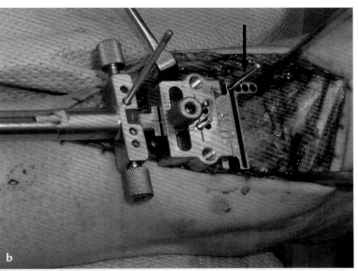

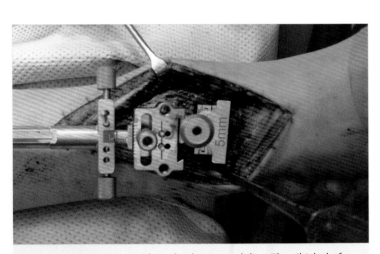

Fig. 6.14 Spacers are used to check joint stability. The tibial platform and spacer are left in place and the talus resection block, which determines size of the polyethylene insert (here 5 mm), is attached to the spacer plate. The talus is resected at the lower edge of the talus resection block. Realignment is carried out in the neutral position with toes pointed toward the ceiling; it may be possible to balance the ligament apparatus over the cut bone surfaces.

Fig. 6.13 (a,b) Positioning of the external tibial alignment guide. Fixation is performed with 2.5-mm pins. The overall approach is very dependent upon the implant. In addition, 0° and 50° resection guide blocks are available for the tibial joint osteotomy. The size of the tibial cutting guide is determined preoperatively. The orientation is verified and the resection is performed approximately 4 mm lower than the deepest portion of the tibial joint surface. A bone pin is inserted to protect the medial malleolus (arrow). The malleoli are at particular risk in rheumatoid patients. The cut must only be directed posteriorly in order to protect the malleoli; the saw should not be allowed to move medially or laterally. The alignment block is aligned with the ankle in the neutral position and toes pointed toward the ceiling. Small imbalances of the ligament apparatus can be corrected by using the tibial and talar osteotomy planes to balance the joint.

6

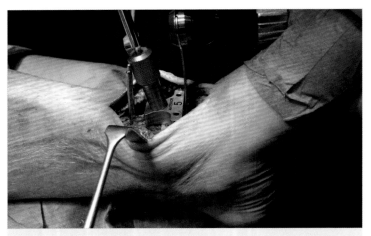

Fig. 6.15 The size of the talar implant is determined. The talar reaming guide is then fastened and the talus surface is prepared. The first talus cut resects the talar dome. An extensive posterior arthrolysis is performed. Resection of the posterior capsule improves posterior extension. A bone or Hintermann distractor is inserted to facilitate the operative procedure.

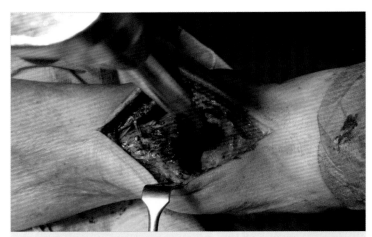

Fig. 6.16 A winged osteotome is used to prepare the talus for the component insertion guide.

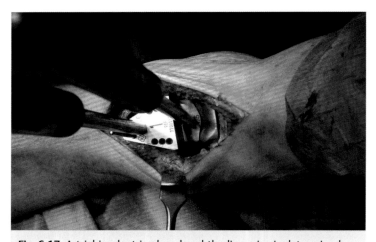

Fig. 6.17 A trial implant is placed and the liner size is determined. Forceful manipulation: the surgeon forcefully performs posterior extension. The remainder of the capsule is disrupted. On rare occasions, an Achilles tendon lengthening is necessary. The lengthening is performed by making three stab incisions on alternating sides approximately 2–3 cm apart. The knife is turned in the middle of the tendon and then guided to the side, thus partially dividing the tendon. Finally, another forceful manipulation is performed. Intraoperative radiographic imaging is necessary to evaluate the position of the implant. The position of the talar dome is assessed in relation to the tibial axis.

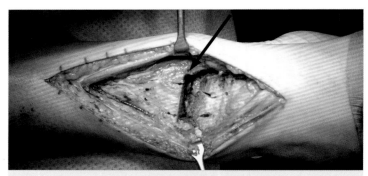

Fig. 6.18 The talus and tibia are prepared. The anchoring site for the medial pin that protects the medial malleolus is easily recognizable.

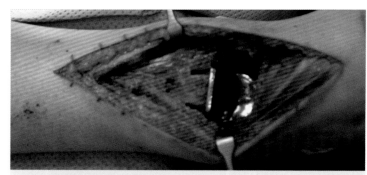

Fig. 6.19 Implanted prosthesis.

6.3 Arthrodesis of the Tibiotalar Joint

▶ **Indication.** Larsen IV–V destruction with significant clinical symptoms. Severe deformity of the tibiotalar joint. Ankle instability. Pronounced bony defects.

▶ **Specific disclosures for patient consent.** Pseudarthrosis. Arthritis in adjacent joints over time. Tendon injury or rupture (also secondary). Bone fracture. Blood vessel and nerve injury. Infection.

▶ **Instruments.** Depending upon the technique:
- Screw fixation, 6.5-mm cancellous screw.
- Plate fixation arthrodesis.
- Intramedullary nail fixation arthrodesis.
- Staple fixation arthrodesis (rare, possibly combined with screws).
- External fixator for pseudarthrosis, infections, or complications.

▶ **Position.** Supine. Ankle in neutral position with toes pointed toward the ceiling. It is usually necessary to place a positioning roll under the buttock in order to compensate for external rotation of hip. The ankle joint rests approximately 3 to 5 cm over the end of the table. A contralateral pelvic support and tilting of the table can be used to achieve a better ankle position. A radiograph may be needed.

▶ **Approach.** Depends upon the procedure: midline (isolated arthrodesis of the tibiotalar joint), lateral (combined with subtalar joint arthrodesis), or medial approaches are possible.

The posterior approach is rarely used. An arthroscopically assisted arthrodesis is very rarely appropriate due to the severe inflammatory changes in the tendons and frequent coexisting axial deviation and bone defects.

We primarily use the midline and lateral approaches.

▶ **Anterior midline approach.** Surgical draping that incorporates the knee is important so that the position of the arthrodesis in relation to the ankle and knee joints can be more accurately assessed.

When possible, the medial and lateral malleoli are not osteotomized in order to maintain a solid position for consolidation of the arthrodesis. See also ▶ Fig. 6.20, ▶ Fig. 6.21, ▶ Fig. 6.22, ▶ Fig. 6.23, ▶ Fig. 6.24.

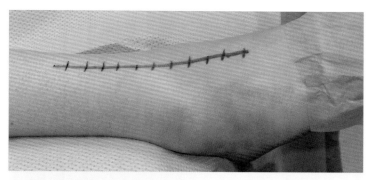

Fig. 6.20 Midline skin incision (a medial or lateral approach also possible).

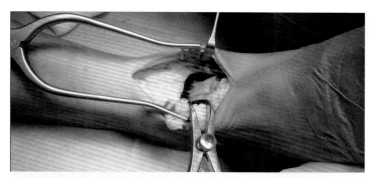

Fig. 6.21 The surgical site is held open with a large spreader. Hohmann elevators are avoided whenever possible, since they often exert excessive pressure on the wound edges and can lead to problems with wound healing. Tibial osteophytes are frequently encountered, and are liberally osteotomized in order to gain a better view of the joint. The joint surfaces are separated with either a bone or Hintermann spreader and then fixed with two K-wires. The cartilage on the joint surfaces is removed with a chisel and Luer. We find the Lexer chisel to be particularly effective. A very sparing bone resection is performed.

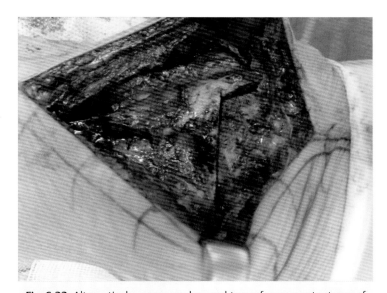

Fig. 6.22 Alternatively, a saw can be used to perform an osteotomy of the joint surfaces.

6

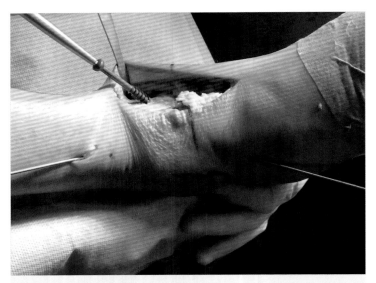

Fig. 6.23 Three K-wires are placed under direct vision, such that the exit point of the wires in the tibiotalar joint can be easily visualized and their potential entry point into the bones on the opposite side can be assessed. The K-wires are not initially drilled over the joint space; this occurs only after all the K-wires have been placed under direct vision and the arthrodesis has been adjusted into the correct alignment. For temporary fixation, we drill a 2.0 K-wire from the heel into the tibia. The arthrodesis position is evaluated in all planes. Next, the screw fitting (normally with three screws) is prepared. Various modifications are possible. Position of screws (our own approach): two screws, one medial and one lateral, are positioned from proximal anterior toward distal posterior. The third screw is inserted into the talus from distal lateral toward proximal dorsal via a stab incision in the tarsal sinus (for screw position, see also ▶ Fig. 6.24). Positioning of the arthrodesis must include the entire portion of the joint that was originally affected, and alignment with the opposite side. The arthrodesis is usually adjusted in a neutral position (up to 5° mild plantar flexion). The hindfoot is held in 5 to 10° valgus, and external rotation is aligned with the opposing side, usually 10°. Only then are the three remaining K-wires pre-drilled.

After placement of the K-wires, intraoperative fluoroscopy is used to assess their position. Then 6.5-mm screws are fitted and drilled over the K-wire. The temporary K-wire through the heel is not removed until all the screws have been placed and viewed under fluoroscopy. For rheumatoid patients, cancellous bone (resected bone, for example) should always be inserted, if possible, in order to improve fusion.

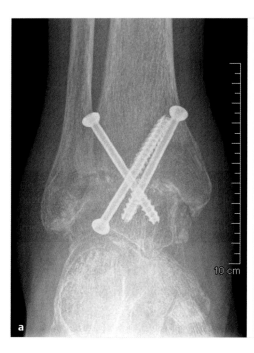
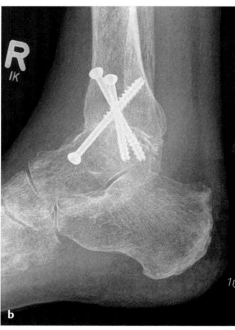

Fig. 6.24 (a,b) Radiographic imaging of the arthrodesis with cannulated screws.

► **Lateral approach.** This alternative approach is particularly used when performing a simultaneous arthrodesis of the subtalar joint. See ► Fig. 6.25, ► Fig. 6.26, ► Fig. 6.27.

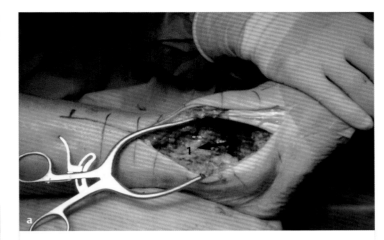

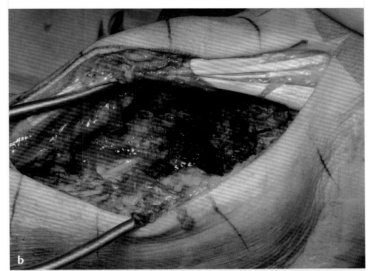

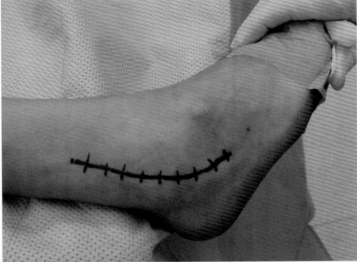

Fig. 6.25 Lateral approach. The incision begins on the anterior edge of the fibula, approximately 5 cm proximal to its tip, and is swung distally over the tarsal sinus. The incision is directed slightly more laterally than the anterolateral standard approach, thus providing better exposure of the subtalar joint.

Fig. 6.27 (a,b) Complete necrosis of talus. The extensor tendons are held off toward midline with a spreader. 1, Tibia. 2, Calcaneus.

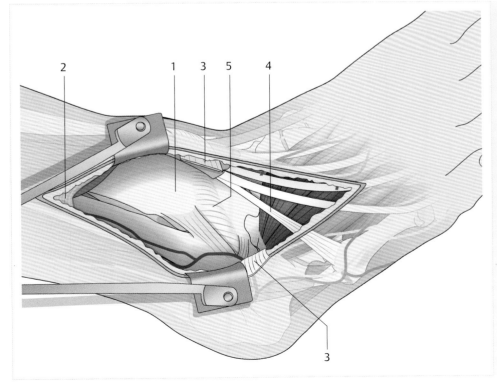

Fig. 6.26 Schematic drawing of the lateral approach. 1, Tibia. 2, Crural fascia. 3, Inferior extensor retinaculum muscle. 4, Peroneus tertius muscle tendon. 5, Talocrural joint capsule.

▶ **Retrograde locking nail osteosynthesis.** See ▶ Fig. 6.28, ▶ Fig. 6.29, ▶ Fig. 6.30, ▶ Fig. 6.31.

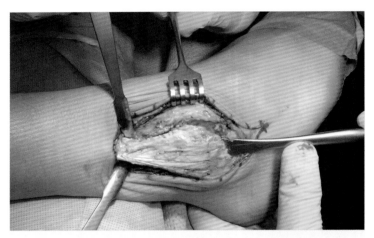

Fig. 6.28 Lateral approach to the ankle joint with an osteotomy of the fibula. This is only performed for extreme preexisting contractures, very severe deformities, or pronounced bone defects because an osteotomy of the fibula reduces the stability of the arthrodesis during the consolidation phase. With retractors under the fibula, an osteotomy is done approximately 6 cm proximal to the fibular tip and the bone is then removed.

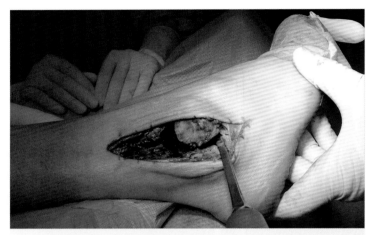

Fig. 6.29 There is now excellent visualization of the ankle and subtalar joint. Cartilage can be removed from all of the joint surfaces. This large incision is very well suited for correction of extreme deformities.

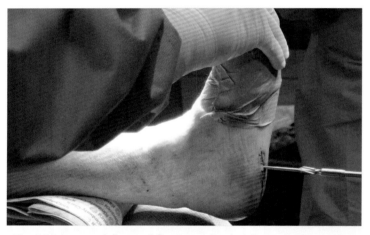

Fig. 6.30 Intramedullary nail fixation arthrodesis/osteosynthesis. The entry point for the drill is imaged in two views under fluoroscopy. An incision approximately 2 to 3 cm long is made, and the tissue is dissected down to the calcaneus. The calcaneus is opened, and the calcaneal entry point is again viewed under radiographic imaging. The guide wire can be advanced through the upper and lower portions of the ankle joint under imaging. Intraoperative radiography is used to image the central position of the guide wire. Only then is drilling over the wire and the actual nail insertion performed.

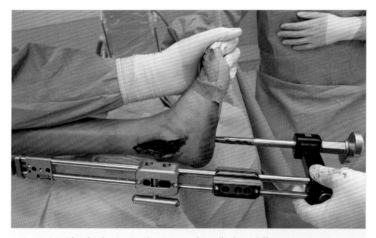

Fig. 6.31 The locking mechanism is handled in different ways depending upon the instrumentation.

▶ **External fixator.** An external fixator can be used for challenging anatomical conditions, extreme contractures, pseudarthroses, and, in particular, for infections.

This technique is often combined with a lateral approach.

The fixator is usually set up in a V-shaped structure: a Steinmann nail in the tibia; a second nail placed in the talus (possibly also calcaneus) posterior to the axis of the tibiotalar joint; the third nail inserted into the talus, anterior to this axis. Depending upon the type of defect, a nail can also be inserted into the midfoot. The nails are inserted from medial toward lateral, so that the tip of the nail is heading lateral and therefore will not lead to injury. With this configuration, uniform compression of the arthrodesis can then be achieved. See also ▶ Fig. 6.32, ▶ Fig. 6.33.

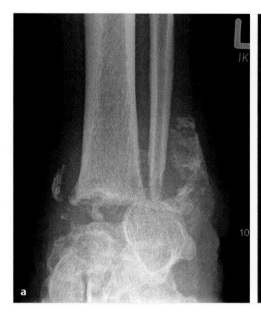 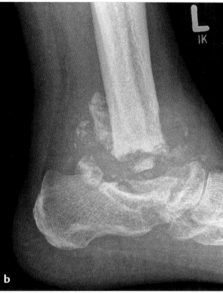

Fig. 6.32 Complete necrosis of the talus bone and partial necrosis of the tibia and calcaneus bone in mutilating rheumatoid arthritis. **(a)** AP radiograph. **(b)** Lateral radiograph.

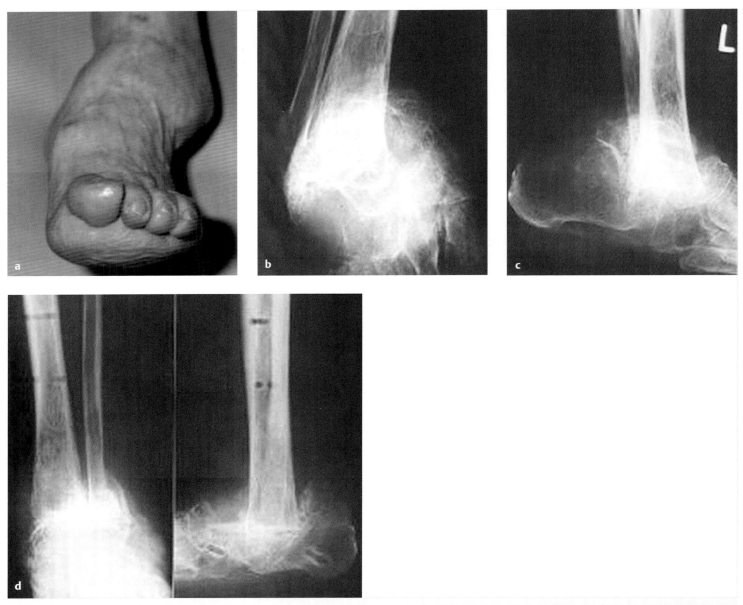

Fig. 6.33 (a–d) Status post fixation procedure. The positions of the Steinman nails can be seen clearly. The lower pin holes show that the bone obviously gave way under the pressure of the nails. This underscores the importance of re-tightening the external fixator in rheumatoid patients.

▶ **Postoperative aftercare.** Depending upon the stability of the osteosynthesis, a stability shoe (VACOped, for example) or a cast boot is used for immobilization. Mobilization without load for the first 6 weeks. After this, radiographic imaging followed by full weight bearing and repeat radiographic imaging prior to clearing the arthrodesis.

The external fixator must constantly be re-tightened, since the rheumatic bone frequently gives way leading to a loss of the compression on the arthrodesis. Re-tightening intervals for the external fixator are after 2 weeks and 6 weeks.

6.4 Arthrodesis of the Subtalar Joint

6.4.1 Arthrodesis of the Talocalcaneal Joint

▶ **Indication.** Larsen III–V destruction. Severe malposition. Bone defects. Clinical symptoms frequently worse than radiologic findings.

▶ **Specific disclosures for patient consent.** Pseudarthrosis. Tendon injury or rupture (also secondary). Bone fracture. Injury to blood vessels and nerves. Infection.

Valgus deformity: it is usually possible to realign by mobilizing the talus from the medial side.

For severe contractures or bone defects: realign with a lateral corticocancellous bone block fusion.

▶ **Instruments.** Depends upon technique; 6.5-mm cannulated cancellous screws. Rarely, staple fixation osteosynthesis.

▶ **Position.** Supine. Ankle in neutral position with toes pointed toward the ceiling. It is usually necessary to place a positioning roll under the buttock in order to compensate for external rotation of hip. The ankle joint rests approximately 3 to 5 cm over the end of the table. A radiograph may be needed.

▶ **Approach.** See ▶ Fig. 6.34.

▶ **Surgical technique.** See ▶ Fig. 6.35, ▶ Fig. 6.36, ▶ Fig. 6.37, ▶ Fig. 6.38, ▶ Fig. 6.39, ▶ Fig. 6.40, ▶ Fig. 6.41.

▶ **Postoperative aftercare.** Depending upon the stability of the arthrodesis, a stability shoe or a cast is used. Mobilization without load for the first 6 weeks. After this, radiographic imaging followed by full weight bearing and repeat radiographic imaging prior to clearing the arthrodesis.

6

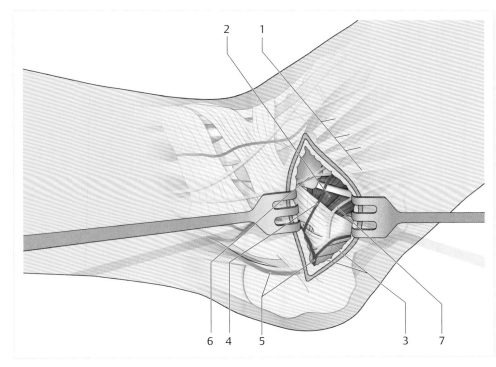

Fig. 6.34 Schematic drawing of the approach. The tarsal sinus is easy to palpate. The incision is made posterior to the middle of the external malleolar tip and extended anteriorly approximately 3 cm. 1, Extensor digitorum longus muscle tendon. 2, Extensor digitorum brevis muscle. 3, Peroneus longus and brevis muscle tendons. 4, Dorsal venous network of foot. 5, Lesser saphenous vein. 6, Intermediate dorsal cutaneous nerve. 7, Lateral dorsal cutaneous nerve (sural nerve).

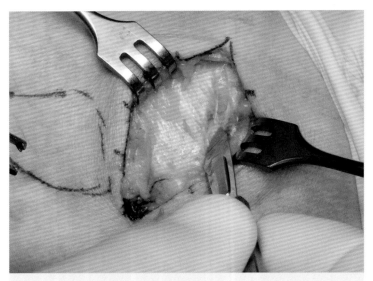

Fig. 6.35 The fascia is divided. The anterior intermediate dorsal cutaneous nerve and the posterior sural nerve must be protected. The inferior extensor retinaculum muscle is divided, and the tarsal sinus, which is easily palpable, is opened.

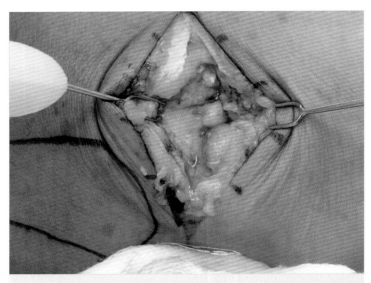

Fig. 6.36 Obvious synovitis in subtalar joint. This is synovectomized with a Luer.

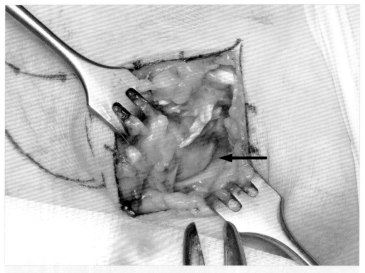

Fig. 6.37 The posterior section of the subtalar joint (arrow) is easy to recognize.

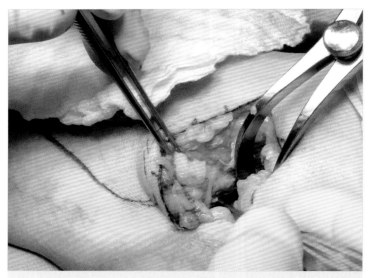

Fig. 6.38 First, a bone distractor is placed into the tarsal sinus. Alternatively, a Hintermann spreader can be used.

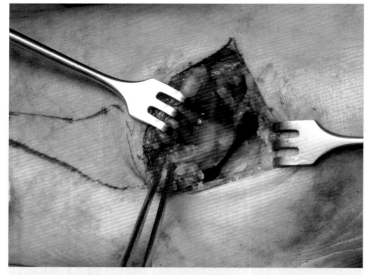

Fig. 6.39 Cartilage is resected from the anterior and posterior section of the subtalar joint (exposed).

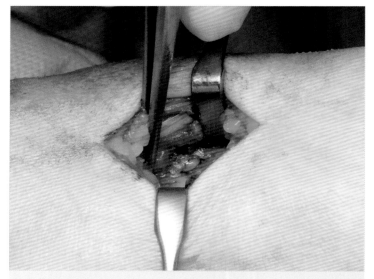

Fig. 6.40 Medially, an incision of approximately 1 cm is made over the talar neck and the tissue is spread with small retractors. The talar neck is exposed and the fixation screws are positioned.

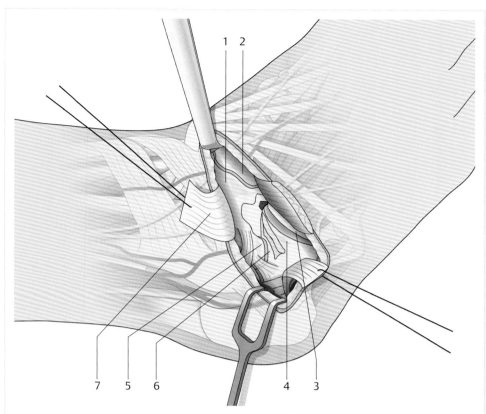

Fig. 6.41 Schematic drawing. 1, Head of talus. 2, Navicular bone. 3, Cuboid bone. 4, Cuboidal articular surface of the calcaneus. 5, Lateral process of talus. 6, Talar articular surface of the posterior calcaneus. 7, Inferior extensor retinaculum muscle.

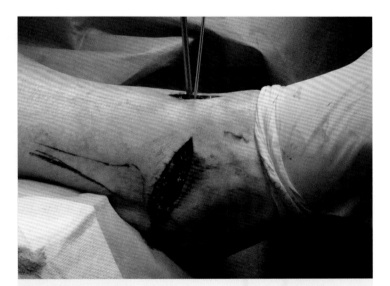

Fig. 6.42 Two K-wires are inserted. The posterior, flatter wire can usually be inserted into the tarsal sinus under direct vision.

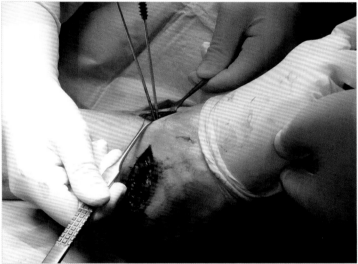

Fig. 6.43 Following fluoroscopic imaging, the K-wires are drilled further. An osteosynthesis is performed.

A classic medial approach to the talus is necessary if the deformity is pronounced (see Chapter 6.4.2). In this case the incision is preferably placed 1 cm more medial and caudal, in order to achieve better mobilization of the talus from the plantar side. The talus is then mobilized completely by performing a medial and lateral release, which returns it to its primary position.

If the deformity cannot be completely realigned, a lateral bone block must also be inserted. See ► Fig. 6.42, ► Fig. 6.43, ► Fig. 6.44, ► Fig. 6.45.

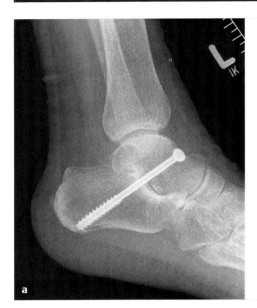

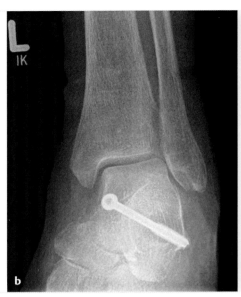

Fig. 6.44 (a,b) The arthrodesis can also be performed using only one 6.5-mm screw.

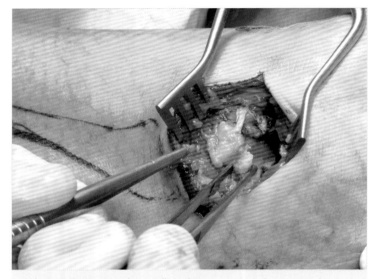

Fig. 6.45 The resected cancellous bone is inserted. In case of persistent valgus deformity, a conforming corticocancellous block is inserted. The screws are aligned and fastened.

6.4.2 Arthrodesis of the Talonavicular Joint

▶ **Indication.** Larsen III–V destruction.

Rheumatic illnesses frequently exhibit involvement of the ankle joint. Clinical symptoms are typically worse than radiologic findings.

▶ **Specific disclosures for patient consent.** Pseudarthrosis. Cancellous bone grafting or a corticocancellous block is necessary for severe bone alignment defects. Infection. Tendon injury. Nerve, blood vessel injury.

▶ **Instruments.** Dependent upon technique: cannulated cancellous screws, 4.5-mm, and/or compression staples.

▶ **Position.** Supine. Ankle in neutral position with toes pointed toward the ceiling. It is usually necessary to place a positioning roll under the buttock in order to compensate for external rotation of hip. The ankle joint rests ca. 3 to 5 cm over the end of the table. A radiograph may be needed.

▶ **Surgical technique.** See ▶ Fig. 6.46, ▶ Fig. 6.47, ▶ Fig. 6.48, ▶ Fig. 6.49.

▶ **Alternatives.** Two cannulated 4.5-mm screws can be inserted. Two K-wires are placed into the navicular bone under direct vision. Once the exit point in the joint surface of the bone is set, the wires are drilled further into the talus bone under direct vision. Following radiographic imaging in two planes, cannulated screws are drilled over the wires.

▶ **Postoperative aftercare.** Depending upon the stability of the arthrodesis, a stability shoe or a cast is used. Mobilization without load for the first 6 weeks. After this, radiographic imaging followed by full weight bearing and repeat radiographic imaging prior to clearing the arthrodesis.

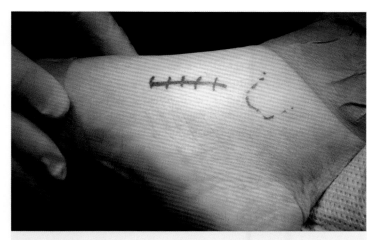

Fig. 6.46 Medial skin incision. The talonavicular joint is usually easy to palpate. In order to mobilize the talus bone for talocalcaneal arthrolysis, the incision is made further plantar. The incision should not be extended posteriorly over the medial malleolus.

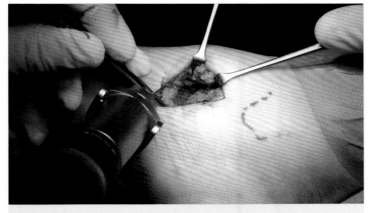

Fig. 6.47 The tibial muscle is preserved. The talonavicular joint is synovectomized and exposed in its entirety. If the defect is not yet pronounced, an attempt should be made to preserve the curved shape of the joint while resecting the cartilage. This is usually easily done using a curved Lexer chisel.

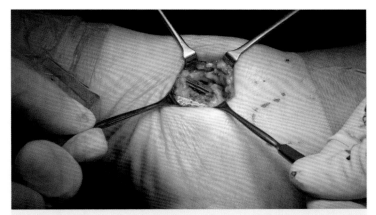

Fig. 6.48 Staple osteosynthesis with 2 to 3-mm staples, which can be inserted under compression.

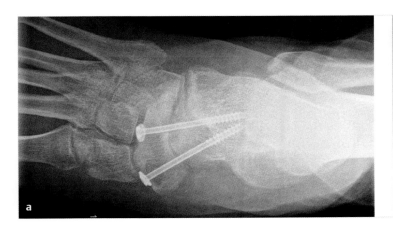

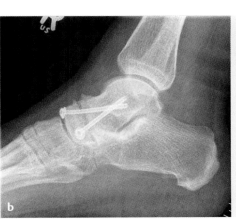

Fig. 6.49 (a,b) Screw fixation osteosynthesis of the talonavicular joint.

Chapter 7

The Knee

7

7 The Knee

S. Sell, S. Rehart, V. Crnic, A. Schoeniger

7.1 Arthroscopic Synovectomy / Baker's Cyst

▶ **Indication.** Larsen 0–III destruction. There must be no significant knee joint instability.

▶ **Specific disclosures for patient consent.** Recurrence. Infection.

▶ **Position.** The Baker's cyst is usually excised first with the patient secured in the lateral position with two pelvic supports. Tilting the table and internally rotating the knee provides a good starting position for a posterior approach to the knee joint.

The pelvic supports are removed following the extirpation, and the patient is turned supine. Arthroscopic synovectomy can then be performed using the same drapes.

▶ **Specifics.** Preoperative ultrasound of the popliteal fossa (on the day before surgery) to determine the cyst dimensions (▶ Fig. 7.1).

▶ **Surgical technique**

▶ **Baker's cyst extirpation.** Approach, see ▶ Fig. 7.2. Surgical technique, see ▶ Fig. 7.3, ▶ Fig. 7.4.

▶ **Arthroscopic synovectomy.** Approach, see ▶ Fig. 7.5. Surgical technique, see ▶ Fig. 7.6, ▶ Fig. 7.7, ▶ Fig. 7.8, ▶ Fig. 7.9, ▶ Fig. 7.10, ▶ Fig. 7.11, ▶ Fig. 7.12. For clinically significant synovitis, arthroscopic synovectomy is combined with radiosynoviorthesis 6 weeks postoperatively.

▶ **Postoperative aftercare.** As a rule, this procedure is followed by radiosynoviorthesis 6 weeks postoperatively.

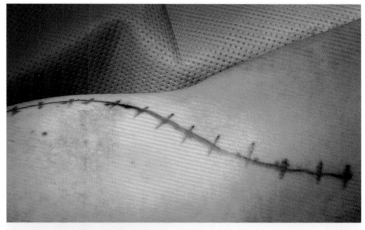

Fig. 7.2 A curvilinear or S-shaped (Trickey's) approach to the Baker's cyst.

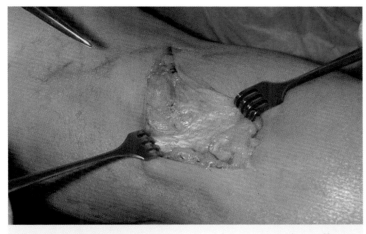

Fig. 7.3 Most often, as in this case, a curvilinear approach is sufficient and can be extended distally if needed. The lower leg fascia is divided.

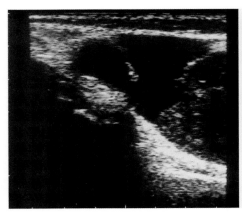

Fig. 7.1 Preoperative ultrasound examination. Multilocular cyst. The exact size of the cyst dictates the size of the incision and can be determined preoperatively.

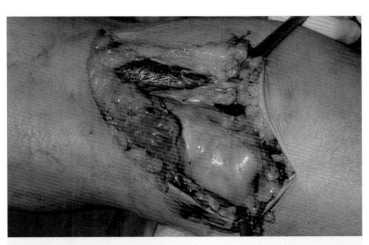

Fig. 7.4 The cyst normally lies between the semimembranosus muscle and the medial head of the gastrocnemius. A large multilocular cyst is pictured. These can usually be detached by blunt dissection with scissors. Better visualization of very large cysts can be achieved by releasing some of the fluid after part of the cyst has been dissected. The stalk connected to the joint is first exposed and then closed.

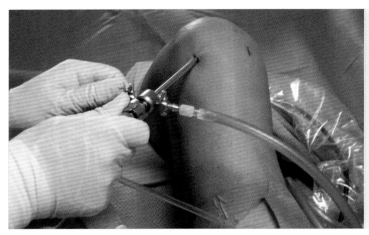

Fig. 7.5 Classic anteromedial and anterolateral approaches. Entry points are frequently made somewhat more proximal than those for a standard arthroscopy. This facilitates a more effective synovectomy of the superior recess, where most of the synovitis masses are commonly located. Synovectomy is performed with a combination of various-sized burs. A vaporizer may be needed for significant bleeding. Two portals are typically sufficient, but more (even dorsal portals) should be used if needed.

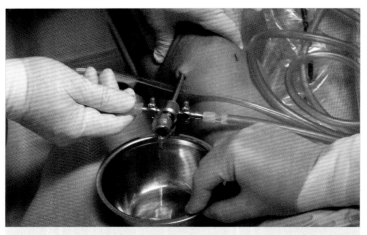

Fig. 7.6 Synovial fluid analysis is always done if there is no definitive diagnosis.

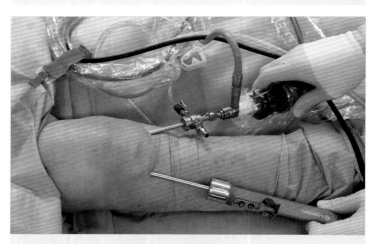

Fig. 7.8 Synovitis in the suprapatellar recess.

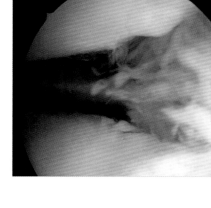

Fig. 7.7 Arthroscopic synovectomy of the suprapatellar recess with the knee in extension.

Fig. 7.9 Pronounced synovitis in the suprapatellar recess.

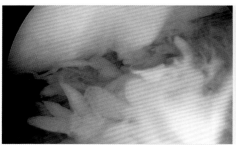

Fig. 7.10 Suprapatellar recess following synovectomy.

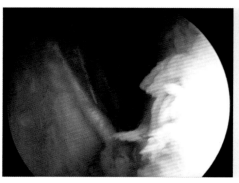

Fig. 7.11 Instruments must be frequently switched between the portals, particularly when performing a synovectomy of the lateral recess.

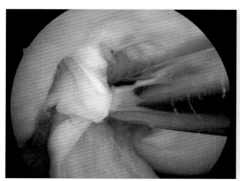

Fig. 7.12 Synovitis around the cruciate ligament is typically removed using small burs.

7.2 Knee Endoprosthesis

Total knee replacement is one of the most common procedures in rheumatoid patients. The knee joint is affected in 90% of patients.

▶ **Indication.** Larsen III–V destruction with significant clinical symptoms.

▶ **Principles for determining treatment.** Treatment is initiated in rheumatoid patients earlier than in osteoarthritis patients. This lessens the likelihood of having to treat multiple joints simultaneously in progressive forms, and thereby avoids the lengthy phases of treatment needed to restore mobility.

Regular and relatively close clinical and radiologic monitoring is important if surgical intervention is deferred for a rapidly progressive inflammatory form. It is not uncommon for these progressive forms to develop significant bone degeneration in the space of 3 to 6 months. This significantly worsens the underlying conditions requiring surgical correction. It is also essential to monitor the supporting ligaments. Progressive laxity of the medial collateral ligament poses a difficult problem surgically, particularly in a knee with valgus deformity.

A highly individualized approach is needed when determining indications for endoprosthesis placement in the lower extremities. Certain basic principles, however, have proved successful:

- Reconstruction of a knee and hip on the same extremity in order to achieve a strong functional leg.
- Proximal before distal: frequently the hips are replaced first.
- For significant flexion contracture of the knee and hip, evidence suggests that it is necessary to address the other ipsilateral joint within a very short period of time so as to avoid the formation of a fixed flexion contracture postoperatively.

In specific situations (such as rapid deterioration of multiple joints), unilateral procedures on multiple joints are possible.

▶ **Specific disclosures for patient consent.** Prosthetic loosening. Bone fracture/perforation. Approximately 3-fold increase in risk of infection. Skin injury (steroid atrophy).

▶ **Instruments.** Prosthesis system from the manufacturer of choice. Uncoupled (cruciate retaining [CR], anterior stabilized [AS], posterior stabilized [PS]), partially coupled, coupled.

▶ **Position.** Supine. Leg holder or sandbag with leg support. A radiograph may be needed.

▶ **Surgical technique**

▶ **Synovitis.** See ▶ Fig. 7.13, ▶ Fig. 7.14, ▶ Fig. 7.15.

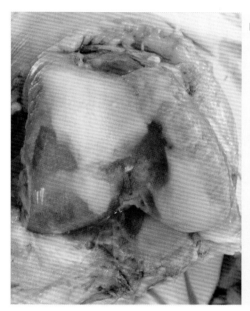

Fig. 7.14 Ochronosis.

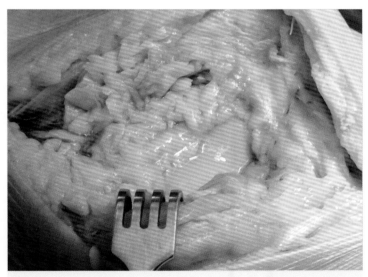

Fig. 7.13 Massive synovitis requires synovectomy of the entire joint. This includes the suprapatellar recess, the medial and lateral compartments, and behind the collateral ligaments. A posterior synovectomy is performed after tibial resection and dissection of the femoral areas. Meticulous hemostasis is vital. Synovectomy should not be performed for inactive synovium because of the potential for fibrosis.

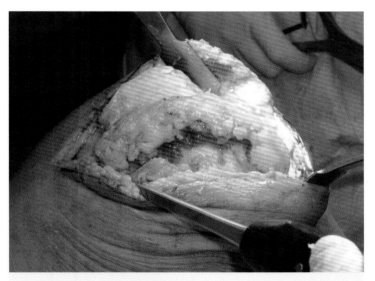

Fig. 7.15 Severe osteophyte formation. All osteophytes should be removed. There are varying forms of disease progression, ranging from minimal to prolific osteophyte formation. Heavy osteophyte production is very common in spondyloarthritis. It is important to be very conscientious about the aftercare of these patients as their knees often stiffen progressively.

▸ **Posterior cruciate ligament (PCL).** There are no general guidelines as to whether the PCL should be resected or preserved. This ultimately depends upon the operative findings.

▸ **Alignment of the components.** Rotational alignment is commonly complicated by considerable bone destruction that is found in a number of rheumatoid patients.

Femoral components: Rotational adjustments are made using multiple reference lines simultaneously. See also ▸ Fig. 7.16.

Valgus deformities of up to 20° are often associated with a 5° external rotation with respect to the dorsal femoral condyles. This external rotation can also be significantly greater in more severe deformities. See ▸ Fig. 7.17, ▸ Fig. 7.18, ▸ Fig. 7.19.

Tibial components: In rheumatoid patients, a functional alignment is used for the tibial component. Following implantation of the trial component, the knee is fully mobilized and the position marked.

In addition, an anatomical alignment is carried out based on anatomical landmarks: using the middle of the tibial prosthesis at the junction of the middle third of the patellar ligament as a guide, externally rotate toward the posterior margin of the tibial plateau.

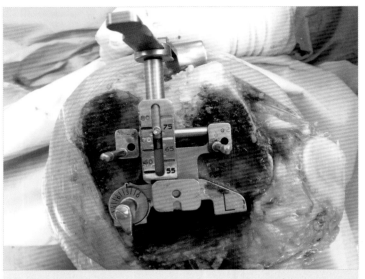

Fig. 7.16 Rotational alignment using the posterior condyles is particularly difficult in valgus destruction associated with destroyed or hypoplastic lateral condyles. In this case the placement of the reference guide must be accurately evaluated to ensure that it is far enough posterior. Otherwise, there is a risk of internal rotation of the femoral component. Bone destruction and missing cartilage lining must be taken into account when comparing and calculating the rotation for alignment.

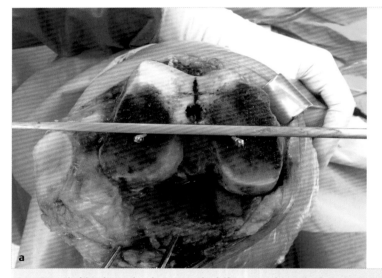

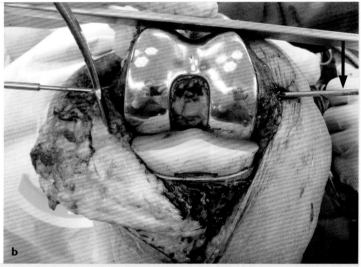

a

b

Fig. 7.17 (a,b) Whiteside's line is marked (for example, with electrocautery) after the joint is opened and before any bone resection. The projected rotation alignment is produced with a chisel by rotating the components after the anchor holes are drilled. In this manner, it can be easily assessed with respect to the Whiteside's line. The epicondyle axis (**b**) is frequently very difficult to palpate, particularly when the destruction is severe. We therefore often alter our surgical procedure for a severe valgus knee deformity: the tibia is osteotomized first, and is then reconstructed. For difficult femoral anatomical landmarks, rotational alignment of the femur is based on the tibia with the aid of the reference lines: Whiteside's line, epicondyle axis, line of the dorsal condyles.

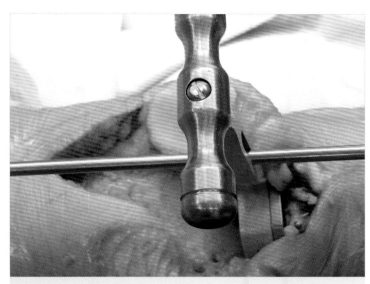

Fig. 7.18 Spacers are used for alignment following tibial resection.

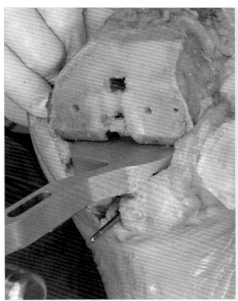

Fig. 7.19 After obtaining sufficient alignment in extension, the flexion gap is adjusted by performing additional dissection of the femoral condyle. Spacers are used to assess the rotational alignment in flexion as well.

▶ **Aligning.** Knee prostheses are implanted with stronger fixation in rheumatoid patients than in osteoarthritis patients. Our experience has shown that knee prostheses have a tendency to loosen again after 5 to 7 years in patients with inflammatory disease. The opposite is true, however, for men with spondyloarthritis. They tend to develop stiffness in the affected knee joint and, therefore, their ligaments should never be tightened excessively during the procedure.

▶ **Rheumatoid valgus knee deformity.** Rheumatoid valgus knee deformity is more difficult to address than varus deformity.

▶ **Classification of valgus knee deformity**
- Grade I: mild valgus deformity. Stable medial ligament. Synovectomy of the knee joint. Standard approach.
- Grade II: lateral contracture, medially still stable. A release of the lateral contracted elements is essential. Testing is performed in both flexion and extension.
- Grade III: severe lateral contracture.
- Grade IIIa: medial laxity, can be realigned (usually up to approximately 40° deformity under load). Intraoperatively, the femoral and tibial weight-bearing surfaces are first resected. Next, spacers are placed, and the knee is initially released in extension. A coupled prosthesis is used if the knee cannot be adequately aligned in extension.
- Grade IIIb: severe medial laxity.
- Grade IV: severe medial and lateral laxity.

A coupled prosthesis is specifically indicated in patients with rapidly progressive and highly inflammatory forms. Approximately 1 to 2% of rheumatoid knee joints fall into this category.

▶ **Realigning the contracted lateral structures.** Extension contracture: the flexion gap is expanded with a bent Hohmann retractor with the knee placed in flexion. The osteophytes are removed by keeping the osteotome continually aimed toward the bone and as perpendicular to the femur as possible. The posterior capsule is elevated off the femur and pushed proximal with a curved rasp. See ▶ Fig. 7.20 for alternative.

7

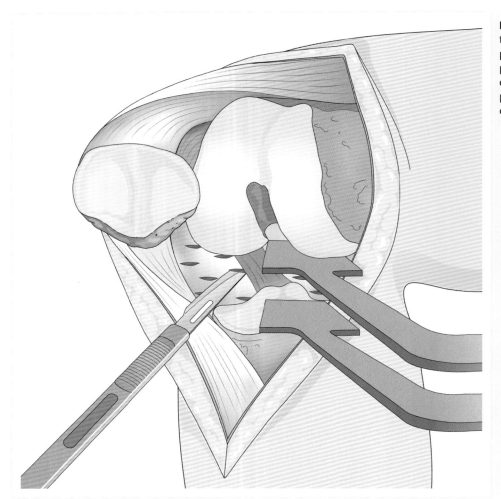

Fig. 7.20 Aligning the contracted lateral structures. As an alternative: The posterior capsule is perforated with stab incisions and then expanded by applying pressure using a Hohmann elevator. Care should be taken around the peroneal nerve, particular with a valgus knee deformity.

▶ **Iliotibial band.** The iliotibial band is dissected extra-articularly. This is accomplished by identifying and exposing the iliotibial band extra-articularly at the level of the joint. The most severely contracted fibers are palpated and released with stab incisions. The tract is then manually stretched. This is repeated until adequate alignment is achieved.

Alternatively, the tract can be exposed intra-articularly; however, the operative view is significantly reduced, so much so that we use this approach only for mild contractures. See also ▶ Fig. 7.21.

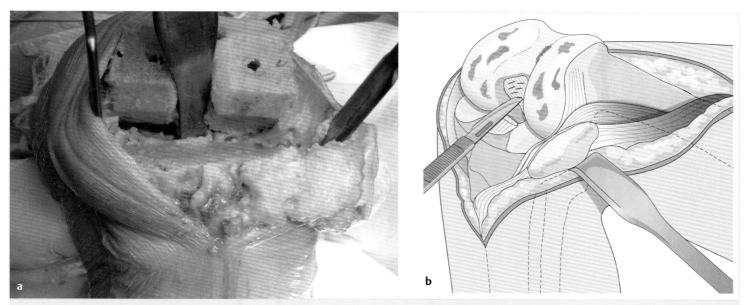

Fig. 7.21 (a,b) Aligning the contracted lateral structures. Flexion contracture: First the tension of the posterior cruciate ligament is examined. If it is contracted, it is carefully incised along the posterior edge of the tibia and stripped off. The ligament is then checked for residual tension. Alternatively, it can be punctured with sharp scissors (see approach for posterior capsule (p. 125)). If contracture persists, the ligament is completely severed. This can result in a 1 to 4-mm expansion of the flexion gap.

If an underlying lateral contracture persists, and the situation warrants, the popliteal tendon is then released.

The lateral ligament is addressed next. An initial release is performed by making stab incisions with subsequent re-expansion.

If this is not adequate, the ligament itself can be released or the bones can be osteotomized and subsequently refixed. The latter, however, requires that the remaining joint stabilizers be of sufficient caliber.

▶ **Rheumatoid varus knee deformity.** Rheumatoid varus knee deformity with medial ligament contracture is less common. See ▶ Fig. 7.22.

▶ **Anchoring.** Bone cement should be used for fixation of prosthesis components because most patients have preexisting osteopenia.

For severe osteoporosis, the shaft of the tibial component is cemented. If necessary, the stability of the entire assembly can be increased with a tibial shaft extension. An overall extension of 80 mm is usually adequate, even in complex cases. See ▶ Fig. 7.23.

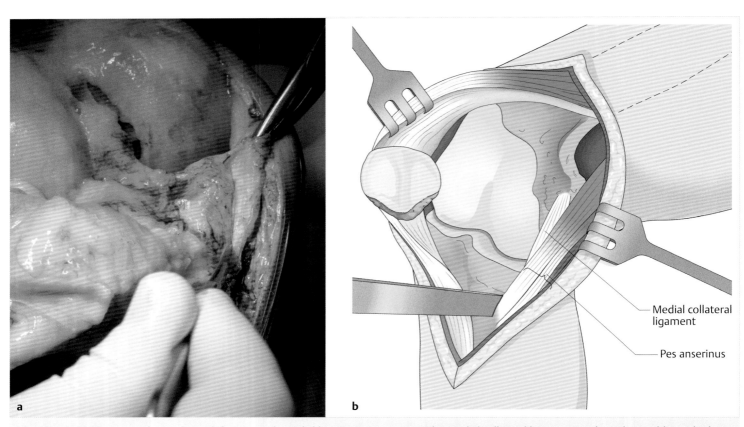

a b

Medial collateral ligament

Pes anserinus

Fig. 7.22 (a,b) Rheumatoid varus knee deformity with medial ligament contracture. The medial collateral ligament is released. An additional release is performed further distally by dividing the pes anserinus from anterior to posterior.

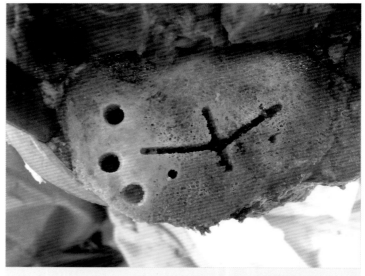

Fig. 7.23 A severely sclerotic tibial plateau can be drilled open for better cementation.

► **Bony defects.** Multiple techniques can be used for reconstruction of tibial defects. Very small, contained defects are filled with cancellous bone or cement. Reconstruction of large defects is often performed with resected bone/transplants taken from the opposite side of the tibia. Augmentations for repair of large defects have also become commonplace. See ► Fig. 7.24, ► Fig. 7.25, ► Fig. 7.26, ► Fig. 7.27, ► Fig. 7.28, ► Fig. 7.29.

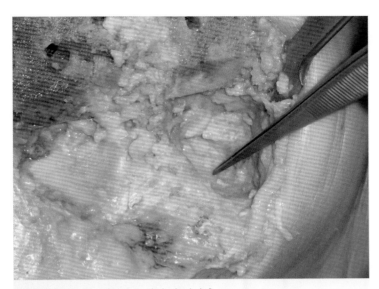

Fig. 7.24 A very deep medial tibial defect.

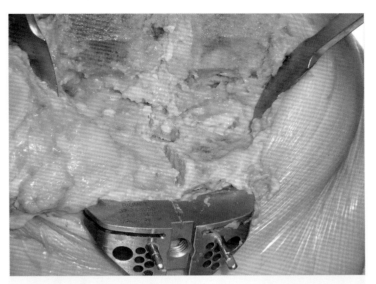

Fig. 7.25 The joint line is first identified on the lateral side and osteotomized accordingly. Further resection is performed on the medial side until the largest part of the defect can be covered with a bone augmentation block.

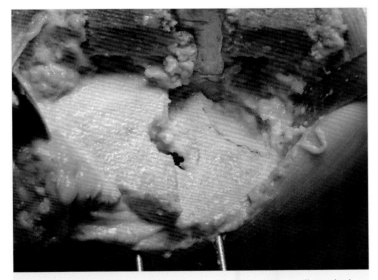

Fig. 7.26 After medial tibial resection, the remaining small residual posterior defect comprises less than one-quarter of the joint surfaces.

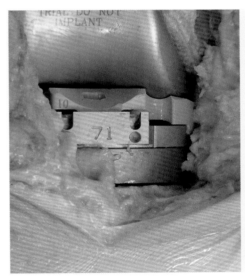

Fig. 7.27 Trial implant with fully balanced medial augmentation block.

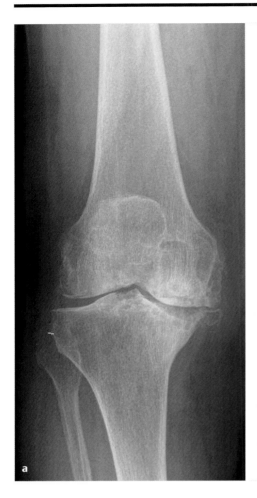

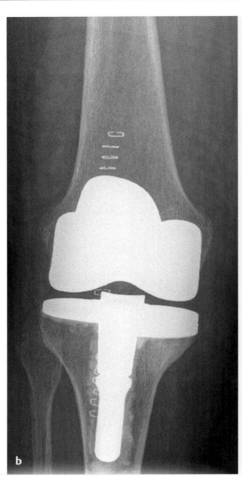

Fig. 7.28 (a,b) A small bony defect.

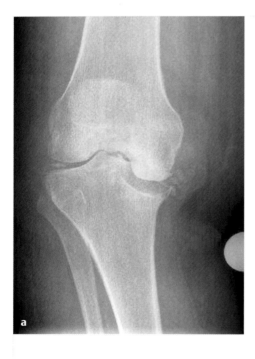

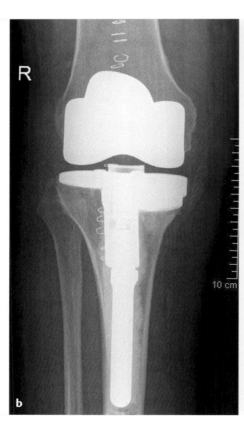

Fig. 7.29 (a,b) Pre- and postoperative radiographs of the affected knee. A large bone defect.

▶ **Complex instability.** See ▶ Fig. 7.30, ▶ Fig. 7.31, ▶ Fig. 7.32, ▶ Fig. 7.33.

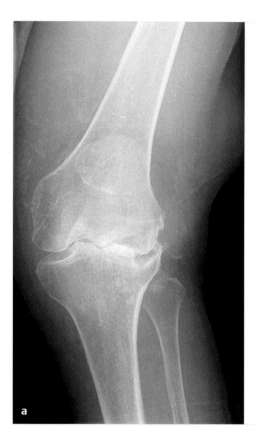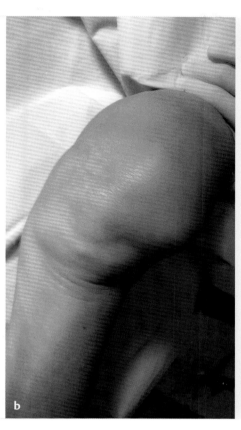

Fig. 7.30 (a,b) Medium-sized bone defect. Clinically pronounced severe medial and lateral instability.

7

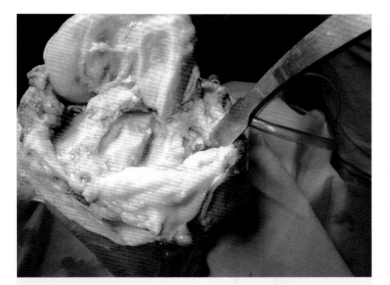

Fig. 7.31 The bone defects appear more significant intraoperatively than on radiographic imaging.

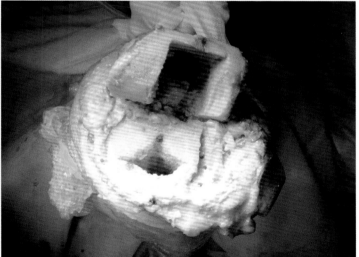

Fig. 7.32 The surgical site after preparation of the prosthesis. The collateral ligaments are resected, and the box cuts are made to preform the femoral site. Any deeper bone defects remaining on the lateral side are perforated with drill holes and sealed with cement.

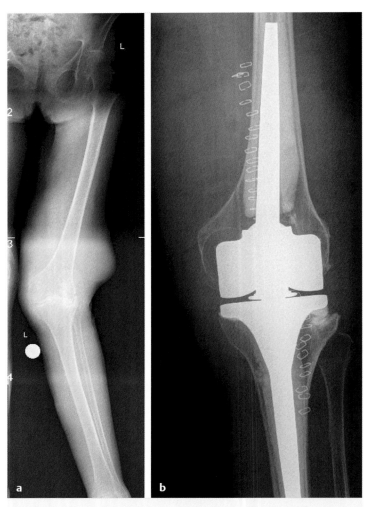

Fig. 7.33 (a,b) Pre- and postoperative radiographs of an affected knee.

▶ **Retropatellar facet replacement.** According to the literature, rheumatoid patients have slightly better clinical results if they also undergo retropatellar facet replacement. For us, the amount of clinical destruction plays an important role in determining surgical indications.

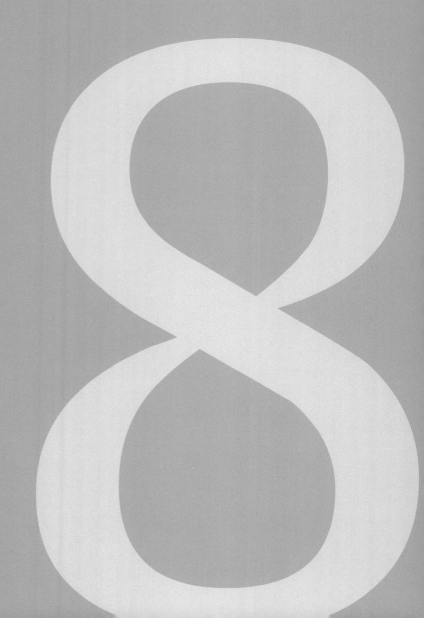

Chapter 8

The Hip

8 The Hip

S. Rehart, S. Sell, V. Crnic, A. Lust

8.1 Hip Prosthesis

▶ **Indication.** Larsen III–V destruction with significant clinical symptoms. Progressive bone destruction, particularly in the acetabular area (acetabular roof necrosis, protrusion, cysts, etc.).

▶ **Principles for determining treatment.** Treatment is initiated earlier in rheumatoid patients than in arthritis patients in order to avoid simultaneous progressive destruction in multiple joints (see also indications for knee prosthesis, Chapter 7.2).

Progressive bone destruction in a rapidly progressing course: do not wait until the acetabular fossa is destroyed. Regular radiographic monitoring is recommended because progression can be relatively asymptomatic compared with the overall level of disease.

▶ **Specific disclosures for patient consent.** Prosthetic loosening; dislocation. Bone fracture; perforation.

▶ **Instruments.** Prosthesis set from the manufacturer of choice.

▶ **Position.** The position will be according to the chosen approach (anterior, anterolateral, dorsal, minimally invasive). The superiority of one approach over another has not been established in rheumatoid patients. It is therefore recommended to use the approach that one is most familiar with. The use of a special hip table is recommended.

▶ **Surgical technique.** See ▶ Fig. 8.1, ▶ Fig. 8.2, ▶ Fig. 8.3, ▶ Fig. 8.4, ▶ Fig. 8.5, ▶ Fig. 8.6, ▶ Fig. 8.7, ▶ Fig. 8.8, ▶ Fig. 8.9, ▶ Fig. 8.10, ▶ Fig. 8.11, ▶ Fig. 8.12, ▶ Fig. 8.13, ▶ Fig. 8.14, ▶ Fig. 8.15.

▶ **Postoperative complications.** See ▶ Fig. 8.16.

Fig. 8.1 A severely obese rheumatoid patient. The bone is frequently very osteoporotic. Traction is placed on the extremity, and the hook is adjusted accordingly. An extensive synovectomy is usually necessary.

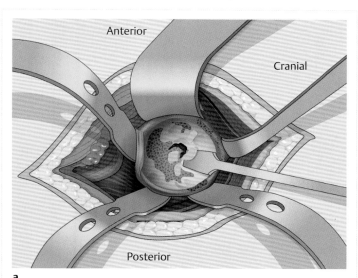

a

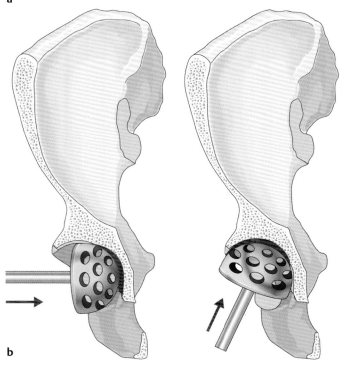

b

Fig. 8.2 (a,b) Exposure of the acetabular lamina interna. Overlying osteophytes may need to be removed with an osteotome. Reaming is initially directed primarily toward the center and then continued in the direction of the acetabular roof. The lamina interna must be reamed under direct visualization because it is very vulnerable if the bone is osteoporotic.

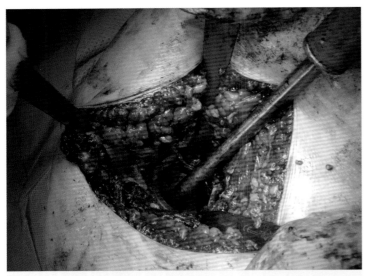

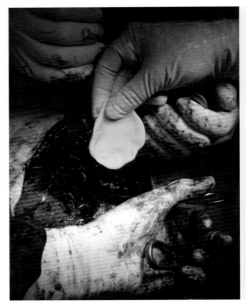

Fig. 8.4 Severely osteoporotic bone requires a cemented socket or an additional acetabular reinforcement cage.

Fig. 8.3 An uncemented press-fit acetabular cup can be anchored even in severely osteoporotic bone. Acetabular impaction bone grafting using the femoral head is also frequently performed. The femoral cancellous bone is placed centrally and compacted with a trial cup.

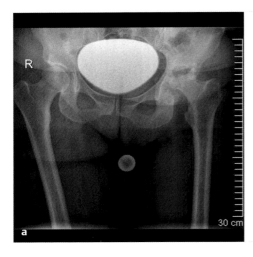

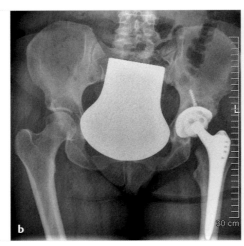

Fig. 8.5 (a,b) Necrosis of the acetabular roof requires careful reaming (also reverse reaming for severely osteoporotic bone). Cancellous bone from the femoral head is used to perform an acetabuloplasty. In poor-quality bone, a rigid fixation is achieved by impacting the press-fit acetabulum and adding screws. An alternative is an acetabular cage with cemented cup.

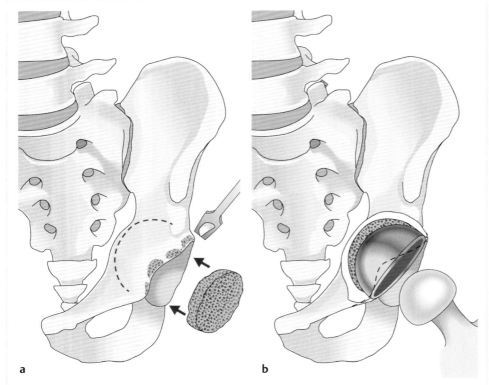

Fig. 8.6 (a,b) For severe protrusion, a wedge of bone is resected from the femoral head and stripped of its cortex. If the bone wedge is too hard, it is weakened by radial incisions made with an osteotome. The graft is placed in the center, impacted with a trial cup, and adjusted so that it lies entirely within the acetabular space.

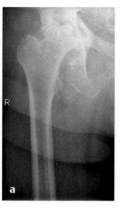
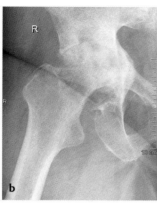
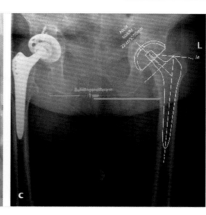

Fig. 8.7 (a–c) Severe acetabular protrusion in rheumatoid arthritis. A cancellous bone wedge is taken from the femoral head and used to reconstruct the acetabular cup.

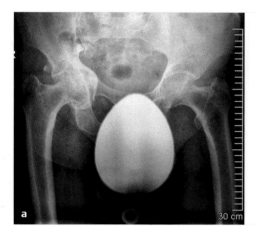
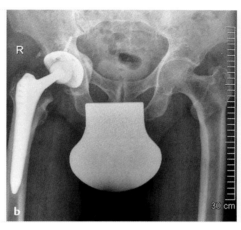

Fig. 8.8 (a,b) Severe acetabular protrusion in ankylosing spondylitis. A bone wedge is removed from the femoral head and used to replace the acetabular floor. The cup is additionally secured with a screw. There is pronounced coxa vara. The center of rotation is realigned by lateralizing the femoral shaft.

8

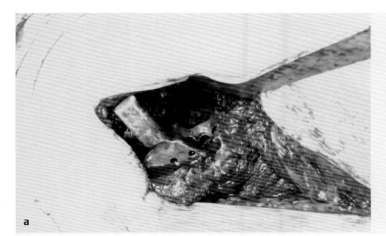
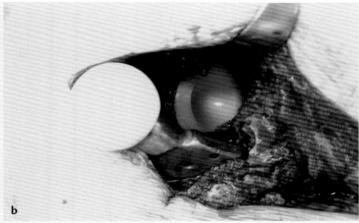

Fig. 8.9 (a,b) Significant protrusion requires an acetabular reinforcement cage and a cup fixed with cement.

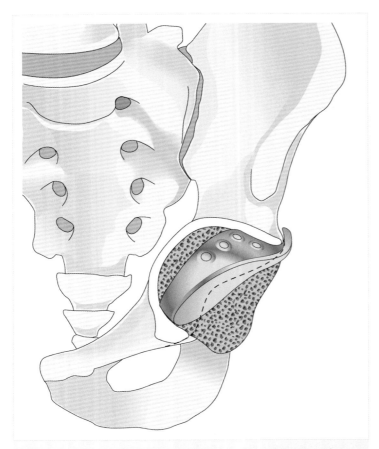

Fig. 8.10 The type of reinforcement cage is dependent upon the amount of protrusion and how reconstructible it is.

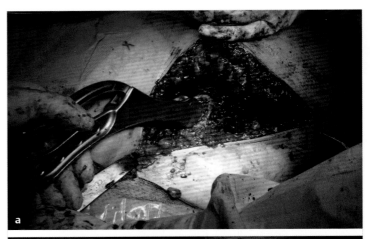

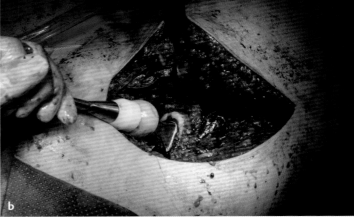

Fig. 8.11 (a,b) Because the bone is often significantly more fragile than suggested on the preoperative radiograph, the soft tissue on the shaft is very carefully exposed and released.

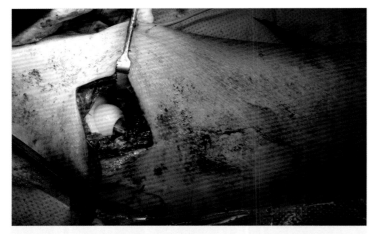

Fig. 8.12 The potential for subluxation and impingement is thoroughly assessed in all directions of movement. In highly inflammatory forms, the periarticular soft tissues are often noticeably elongated.

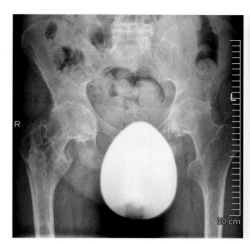

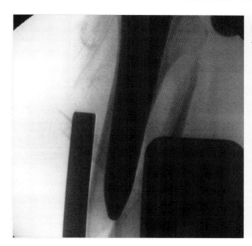

Fig. 8.13 Long-standing rheumatoid arthritis. Severe osteoporosis.

Fig. 8.14 Intraoperative shaft fracture.

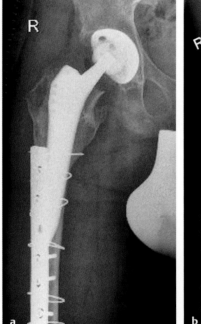

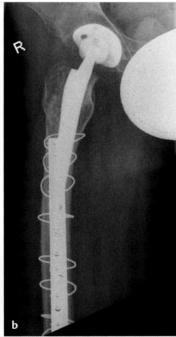

Fig. 8.15 (a,b) Surgical internal fixation.

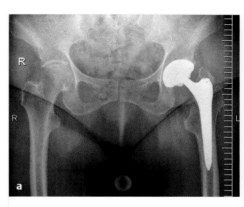

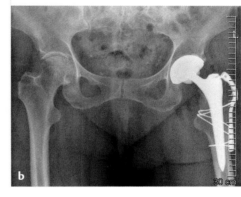

Fig. 8.16 (a,b) Trochanter fracture 8 weeks postoperatively in a patient with long-standing rheumatoid arthritis and long-term cortisone therapy.

8

Chapter 9

The Spine

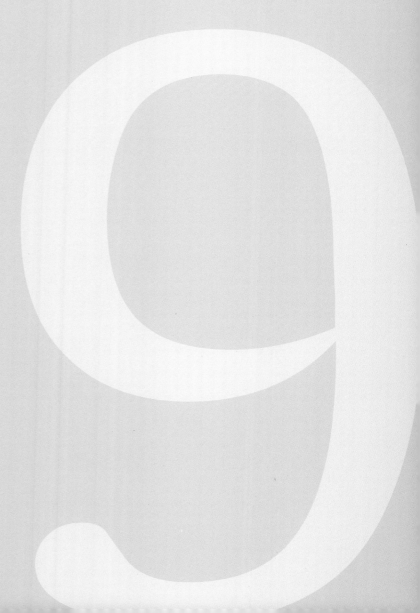

9 The Spine

H. Boehm

9.1 Cervical Spine: Atlantoaxial Reduction and Fusion

▶ **Indication.** Atlantoaxial instability > 5 mm. Significant retrodental pannus formation. Onset of cranial settling.

▶ **Differential therapeutic considerations.** Is there a preexisting fixed dislocation and/or significant cranial settling that requires a transoral odontoid resection and release before the spondylodesis procedure? Is there any pertinent segmental instability that could affect intubation?

▶ **Anesthesia specifics.** Metal-reinforced endotracheal tube. Videolaryngoscopic or fiberoptic intubation. Anesthetic agents must be limited to those that allow for intraoperative neuromonitoring. Anesthetist and anesthesia equipment are positioned at the foot of the patient.

▶ **Specific disclosures for patient consent.** Risk of vertebral artery injury resulting in:
- Ischemic damage in the vascular territory of the basilar artery.
- Significant blood loss.

Proximal spinal cord injury. Occipital nerve injury/neuralgia. Implant malposition with dural injury. Risk of pseudarthrosis and subsequent implant failure.

▶ **Instruments.** Basic dorsal cervical spine pan:
- Open approach: C1–C2 transarticular screw fixation instruments, 2.7-mm or 3.2-mm diameter screws with a length of 38 to 48 mm.
- Mini-open technique: sleeve guide system for percutaneous placement of screws using Magerl's technique.
- As a modification for either of the above, if standard straight instruments cannot be used for a severe high thoracic kyphosis, curved drill sleeves (see ▶ Fig. 9.6) are needed.
- The Harms/Melcher cervical polyaxial screw-rod fixation system (see below) may be needed for C1 and C2 stabilization. An occipital plate is also required if there is advanced C1 destruction.

If a transoral release is necessary, the Crockard or Harms transoral instrument set will be required. Radiologic image intensifier. Intraoperative neuromonitoring. Intraoperative computer-assisted navigation may be needed.

▶ **Preoperative considerations / specific diagnostic investigation.** Assessment of the C1 joints: are they still large enough? If not, C0–C2 fusion using an occipital plate/rod system is indicated.

The extent of thoracic kyphosis and deflectability of the subaxial cervical spine determine whether the orientation for the transarticular drilling and screw placement can be achieved.

Are vertebral arteries present on both sides and is their caliber sufficient?

Is there any alteration in the spatial relationship between axis or atlas and the vertebral arteries as they exit C2 and enter the foramen magnum (▶ Fig. 9.1)? If so, are the vessels at risk of injury after repositioning or during drilling and screw placement?

Is intraoperative spinal cord monitoring necessary?

If functional imaging of the head demonstrates inadequate reducibility in extension, the need for transoral joint mobilization and/or odontoid resection as a preceding step should be determined preoperatively. Usually, however, intraoperative reducibility is significantly greater than that indicated by the preoperative functional imaging.

▶ **Position.** Prone position on a spine frame. Operating table with adjustable head section. Head positioning device, possibly with a mirror that allows for intraoperative assessment of position-related pressure points on the eyes and nose (prone view). The table should be tiltable head up/feet down to reduce blood loss. However, this position requires a mechanism to prevent the patient from shifting caudally.

Sterile draping that allows:
- Radiolucent imaging in two planes.
- Intraoperative adjustability of the headrest for reduction.
- Access to the posterior iliac crest for extraction of a corticocancellous graft.

▶ **Key steps**

▶ **If reducibility is questionable.** Following induction of anesthesia under full muscle relaxation and in supine position, place a strong support underneath the spinous processes from C2 to C7 and apply pressure through the mouth on the anterior arch of C1 under the guidance of lateral fluoroscopy imaging. If not adequately reducible, an additional transoral release should be performed before the posterior fixation/fusion, in order to allow reduction (see below).

▶ **Bone graft harvesting.** It is preferable as the first step to obtain a corticocancellous graft from the posterior iliac crest: A 3-cm-long skin incision is made just lateral to the posterior spine of the iliac crest, and a 15 × 25 × 6 mm corticocancellous wedge is extracted from the outer table. By maintaining meticulous control of the osteotome, the posterior iliac crest and its stability can always be preserved, and injury to the iliosacral joint avoided. Additionally, using a curet, a few cancellous bone chips should be taken, which can later be packed laterally underneath the structural graft. To minimize postoperative blood loss, bleeding bone surfaces are carefully covered with a collagen fleece.

▶ **Approach.** If the open technique is used for transarticular screw fixation of C2/C1, the skin incision must be extended down to the level of the T1 spinous process, and the posterior neck musculature must be deflected down to C6 in order to accommodate the implantation angle. In addition to the tissue trauma of the approach, this increases the risk of secondary muscle dehiscence and impaired wound healing. Intraoperative orientation, accuracy of drilling, and screw placement are slightly more difficult if it is carried out using our mini-open technique. Because drilling and screw implantation are performed percutaneously through drill sleeves inserted into two high thoracic stab incisions, our procedure minimizes the posterior exposure to the area of C1 and C2. The technique is described below.

▶ **Surgical technique for atlantoaxial reduction and fusion.** Make a midline incision 4 cm in length from the occiput to the spinous process of C2, see ▶ Fig. 9.2.

Perform subperiosteal exposure of the C2 spinous process and continue dissecting laterally toward the lamina and the C2–C3 intervertebral joint. This is best accomplished using a Cobb elevator. Countertraction is necessary if there is significant preexisting translational and rotational instability. After palpation of the arch of C1, an additional 15 mm on each side of the midline is exposed subperiosteally. The area cranial to the arch of the atlas should not be exposed further laterally due to its proximity to the vertebral artery. Venous plexuses run in the lateral portion of the C1–C2 interlaminar space (V in ▶ Fig. 9.3) and have a tendency to bleed heavily. As a rule, hemorrhage can be prevented by bluntly separating the soft tissues and pushing them to the side with a small cotton swab.

After determining the insertion point, make an 8-mm stab incision (▶ Fig. 9.4). Introduce the coupled drill sleeve, initially fitted with an awl. Verify the direction and the correct entry point, first in a lateral radiographic view and then in AP. Under fluoroscopic imaging, drill through C2 into the joint space of C2/C1, which usually can be felt. Verify the reduction and continue drilling through C1, aiming at the middle third of the anterior arch under lateral radiographic control. A drill sleeve guide (▶ Fig. 9.5) is useful for this step. Determine the correct screw length. Replace the second drill and inner bushing with a screwdriver and attached screw. Insert a washer into the exposed site and capture it with the tip of a screw that has been inserted through the guide sleeve. Turn the screw under fluoroscopic imaging while maintaining direct visualization of the insertion site and carefully watching for inadvertent C1–C2 joint distraction.

If a sufficiently small angle cannot be maintained due to a high thoracic kyphosis, one solution might be to use the curved drill sleeve system (shown in ▶ Fig. 9.6) instead of the straight sleeve.

Following reduction, the goal is to achieve a bony bridge between the C1 and C2 laminae. This is optimally achieved by bridging with a U-shaped corticocancellous iliac graft that is affixed to the arches of C1 and C2 and the spinous process of C2. The Magerl screw technique generally ensures adequate primary stability of the construct. It is therefore normally sufficient to secure the graft with a nonresorbable no. 2 suture using the Gallie technique, a cost-effective and MRI-compatible solution.

In addition, hypertrophy of the ligamentum flavum may lead to a stenosis between the atlas and axis. To avoid any risk of postoperative stenosis and in order to have optimal visual control during sublaminar placement of the thread, the dura should be dissected free several millimeters on each side of the midline.

The ligaments connecting the occiput and atlas, however, should be weakened as little as possible. Remove a 3-mm-wide section of the atlanto-occipital ligament. This will provide

sufficient space to pull the suture through or, if necessary, to perform a more stable fixation with a cable or wire equivalent. We prefer to use a modified Overholt clamp for passing the thread around the posterior arch of the atlas (▶ Fig. 9.7). The doubled suture is looped around the arch of C1 and can be used for maneuvers of reduction and for temporary fixation to the C2 spinous process during drilling.

Correct placement of the drill hole is crucial for stable and safe screw fixation (see also ▶ Fig. 9.8).

Magerl developed a very efficient technique to determine the mediolateral insertion point by palpating the medial pedicle edge and entering 2 to 3 mm lateral to it. The other coordinate for placement of the screw lies on the C2 joint facet just cranial to its capsular insertion point. See ▶ Fig. 9.9, ▶ Fig. 9.10, ▶ Fig. 9.11.

▶ **Surgical technique for transoral joint release and/or odontoid resection when atlantoaxial subluxation is no longer reducible.** If an attempt at manual realignment under general anesthesia (see above) demonstrates that the subluxation is not adequately reducible, the patient is kept in the supine position and transoral mobilization is carried out prior to posterior stabilization. It is usually insufficient to simply mobilize the atlantoaxial joints because of reactive changes at the atlantodental joint. Therefore, the necessity of an odontoid resection should be included in the preoperative planning and when taking the patient's consent.

To make a monosegmental procedure possible, the anterior arch of the atlas must be preserved. Our own technique is outlined below.

It is best to perform the transoral portion under visualization with an operating microscope, with the surgeon sitting at the patient's head. Following orotracheal intubation, the nasopharyngeal cavity is disinfected with betadine solution (see ▶ Fig. 9.12).

After insertion of a mouth and uvula retractor the anterior tubercle of the atlas is easily palpable, even in rheumatoid patients, and serves as a landmark throughout the procedure. The approach is through a midline incision from the base of C2 up to 1 cm cranial to the anterior tubercle. An adequate exposure and secure wound closure are obtained by sharply detaching the capitus longus muscle transversely from the caudal edge of the arch of the atlas and pushing both the muscle and its mucosa laterally.

Dissecting laterally along the caudal arch of the atlas leads to the C1–C2/C2 joint even in cases of subluxation (▶ Fig. 9.13b). After verifying the position of the vertebral artery, the joint is cleaned out on both sides, and reduction is attempted using an elevator. If this is sufficient, the joint cartilage is completely removed, and the incision is closed. If the correction is inadequate and there is a possibility of (or preoperative diagnostic investigation shows) a substantial retrodental mass, the procedure is expanded to include an odontoid resection (▶ Fig. 9.14, ▶ Fig. 9.15).

The principle of an atlas-sparing odontoid resection consists of making a 5-mm-wide transverse osteotomy on the base of the odontoid and pulling the odontoid peg caudally in a stepwise fashion utilizing a threaded K-wire (▶ Fig. 9.15a).

As soon as the defect of the osteotomy has been closed by this maneuver, a second K-wire is inserted cranial to the first (▶ Fig. 9.15b) and the caudal end of the odontoid is shortened another 5 mm. This step may need to be repeated until the remainder of the odontoid is free and can be removed (▸ Fig. 9.15c). Rarely, the apical odontoid ligament, if still present (uncommon in rheumatoid patients), may need to be cut.

Finally, remove the retrodental granulation tissue. It is not uncommon to find solid masses that have formed from long-standing cysts that have filled with fibrin over time. Caveat: The walls of those cysts can be densely adherent to the dura. See also ▸ Fig. 9.16.

In the last step the detached parts of the longus colli muscle are folded back and reattached. The posterior pharyngeal wall is closed with embedded full-thickness interrupted stitches. The surgeon places a gastric tube through the mouth prior to turning the patient prone for posterior screw fixation and spondylodesis.

▸ **Specific complications.** Implant malposition. Injury to the dura. Pseudarthrosis with secondary implant breakage. Distraction of the C1–C2 joint space

▸ **Postoperative aftercare.** Neck brace for 8 to 12 weeks, depending upon bone quality. Isometric exercises. Patient-driven exercises of the neck muscles against resistance.

In the event of an additional transoral procedure, give parenteral nutrition and antibiotic coverage for the first 5 days; daily antiseptic mouth rinses.

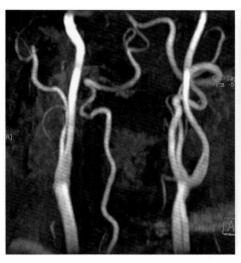
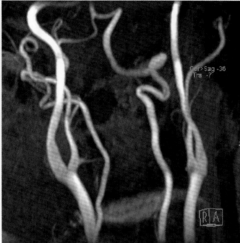

Fig. 9.1 Confirmation that vertebral arteries are present on both sides with a normal anatomical course to the basilar artery

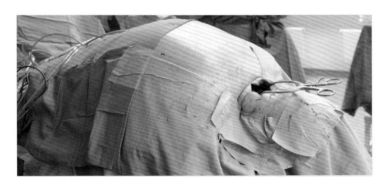

Fig. 9.2 The skin incision is made from the occiput down to the spinous process of C3. The anesthetist is located at the foot end of the table on the right. This allows access to the head, neck, and upper body as well as to the posterior iliac crest for bone graft retrieval.

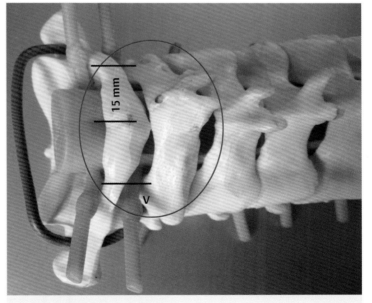

Fig. 9.3 Model of the exposed area: The ellipse indicates the exposed posterior craniocervical junction. Large convoluted veins (V) lie posterior to the root and can lead to significant blood loss.

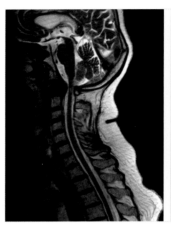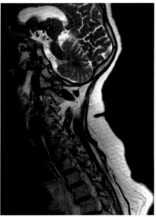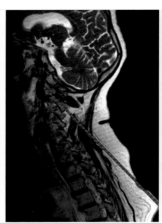

Fig. 9.4 Determine the site for the stab incision that will be used for percutaneous insertion of the drill and screws. The landmarks for drill orientation in relation to the spinous processes can be more easily obtained by comparing the median sagittal scan to one that runs laterally through the joint. The red line indicates the desired entry points at skin and C2. Judge from the sagittal MRI whether cervical hyperlordosis or thoracic hyperkyphosis could hinder screw placement. An axial MRI calculated in the plane of the red line ("Magerl view") indicates where the vertebral artery could be hit.

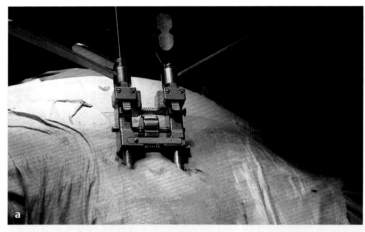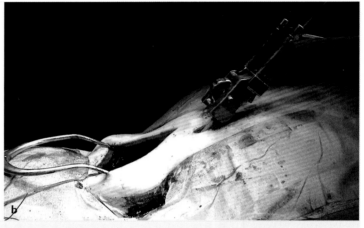

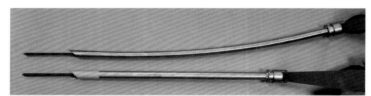

Fig. 9.5 (a) The drill sleeve for percutaneous placement of drill holes and insertion of screws along with the alignment block. The drill on the left side has already been inserted. On the right side, an awl marks the correct insertion point and secures the right side of the drill sleeve. (b) View from the left side: The percutaneous approach nearly halves the length of required spinal column exposure.

Fig. 9.6 Mini-open technique: the sleeve system for drill and screw insertion is pictured. At the top is shown a curved system that can be used when, for anatomical reasons, the optimal angle cannot be obtained with a straight sleeve.

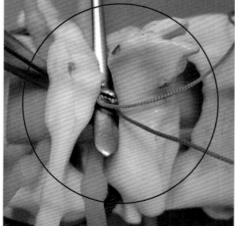

Fig. 9.7 Placement of the graft-fixating suture around the posterior arch. Under constant bony contact a right-angled Overholt clamp is passed from cranial to caudal while protecting the dura at C1–C2. Then a nonresorbable no. 2 suture is grasped midway and pulled through, thus looping around the arch.

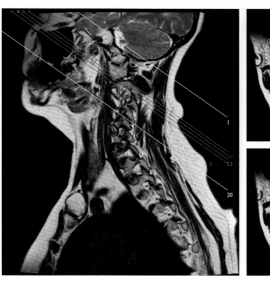
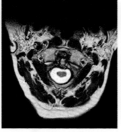
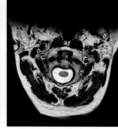
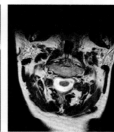

Fig. 9.8 The advantage of "Magerl trajectory imaging." Imaging planes are chosen such that they correspond to the subsequent orientation of the screw. The ideal location for the drill is in slice 10. Upper right is the axial slice (prior to reduction). This permits a continuous bone channel for the screw through C2 and C1. The vertebral arteries can be seen in slices 9 and 12 and are located sufficiently far away. In this case, the anatomical conditions do allow insertion of drills and screws through a small main incision.

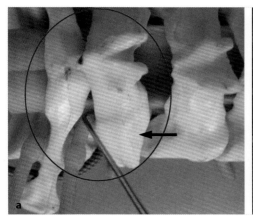
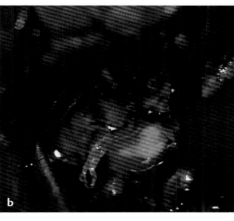

Fig. 9.9 (a,b) A ballpoint hook is used to determine the medial pedicle edge of C2. The entrance point on the C2 facet is opened with a small bur 2 to 3 mm laterally and as caudally as possible.

9

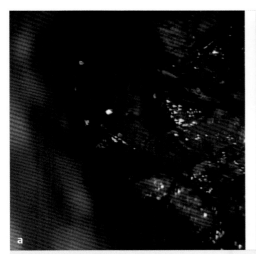
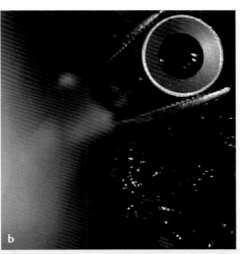
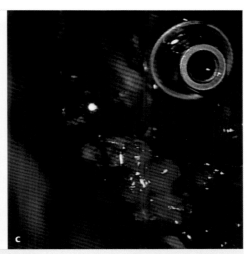

Fig. 9.10 (a–c) The awl from the inserted sleeve system in ▶ Fig. 9.5 is replaced with a drill. Under fluoroscopic imaging in the lateral view, a hole is drilled all the way into the C2–C1 joint **(a)**. Then, by using the sublaminar thread in ▶ Fig. 9.7 and holding the C2 firmly, the atlas is repositioned relative to the axis and held in place while drilling is continued to the anterior cortex of C1. This is performed at a higher drill speed. In addition, care must be taken to ensure that the joint gap does not widen during drilling. After performing the same procedure on the other side, the reduction of C1 on C2 is retained temporarily. The first drill is then replaced with a screw, and after repeating this sequence on the other side definitive fixation is achieved. A washer should be used for osteoporotic bones. It is inserted through the incision **(b)** and then captured and fixated by the screw within the sleeve **(c)**.

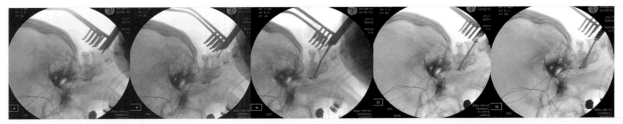

Fig. 9.11 Sequence for the insertion of drill and screws into C2 and C1. Left, the percutaneous drill sleeve has been inserted, and the entry point is enlarged with an awl. The awl is then replaced with the drill, and a second drill hole is placed. The first drill is replaced with a 2.7-mm screw, followed by the second screw through the second drill hole.

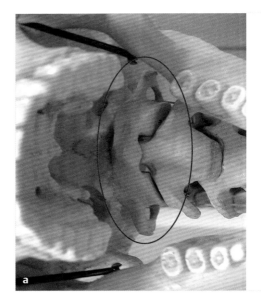

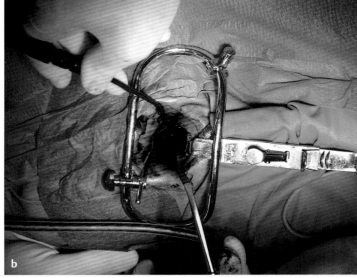

Fig. 9.12 Transoral release including atlas-preserving odontoid resection. (a) In the model: the red oval encircles the field of view, which is held open with a Crockard spreader. (b) Patient with mouth and uvula retractor after sterile draping.

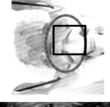
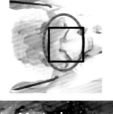
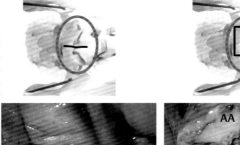

Fig. 9.13 (a) View of the posterior pharynx wall from the patient's right side. The uvula retractor is visible on the left edge of the picture. A midline incision through mucosa and muscularis is visible. (b) The left joint is exposed (J). AA denotes the left side of the arch of the atlas. (c) The base of the odontoid (O) is exposed. The atlantodental joint cartilage emerges cranial to the base.

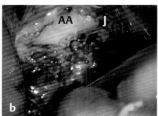
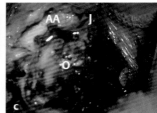
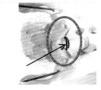
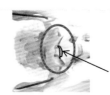
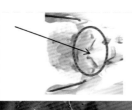
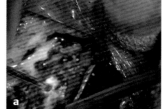
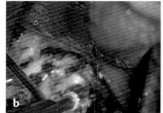
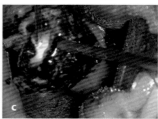

Fig. 9.14 Osteotomy of the odontoid. (a) First, a K-wire with a threaded tip (see the arrow in the schematic) is inserted into the odontoid as far cranial as the preserved arch of C1 allows.
(b) Next, a burr and Kerrison are used to make a 5-mm transverse osteotomy at the base of the odontoid. (c) Osteotomy gap (blue on the model) after complete detachment of the odontoid.

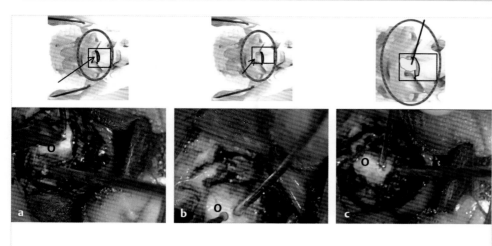

Fig. 9.15 Mobilization and removal of the odontoid. **(a)** The odontoid (O) is pulled down over the fixation wire by deflecting it with a chisel (the arrow on the model). This maneuver partially closes the osteotomy. **(b)** The odontoid is then caudalized as far as possible, thus closing the osteotomy. Next, the insertion site for a second fixation wire is burred open as far cranial as possible. **(c)** The caudal wire has been removed and the odontoid, held by the second K-wire, is shortened caudally with a 5-mm Kerrison and pulled caudally using the maneuver in **(a)** until the osteotomy is closed again. Finally, the remaining cranial part (yellow on the model) of the odontoid is now completely mobile and can be taken out in the next step.

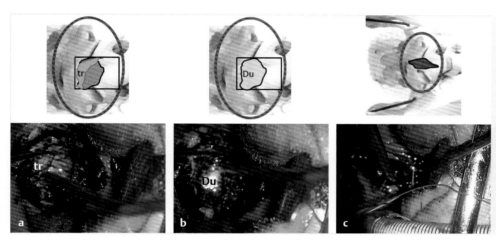

Fig. 9.16 The odontoid has been removed. **(a)** In the retrodental tissue mass a partially preserved transverse ligament (tr; yellow on the model) can be identified. **(b)** The fully decompressed, uninjured dura (Du; blue on the model). **(c)** The posterior pharyngeal wall wound (red area in model) is closed with deep sutures.

9.2 Thoracolumbar Corrective Osteotomy for Ankylosing Spondylitis

▶ **Indication.** Global thoracic and lumbar kyphosis with:
• Significant thoracic or thoracolumbar hyperkyphosis.
• Loss of lumbar lordosis.
• Angular deformity after a healed fracture or an Andersson lesion.

▶ **Differential diagnosis and therapeutic considerations.** Evaluate the deformity to locate optimal correction point(s) and determine the extent of correction needed/desired. In addition, assess the extent and location of the anteriorly fused segments / syndesmophytosis. Depending upon the results, decide whether to perform a pedicle subtraction osteotomy (PSO) or dorsoventrodorsal (minimally invasive) corrective osteotomy.

Other issues to consider are the need for an increased number of fixation points due to poor bone quality; deformity of the cervical spine that may eventually require additional correction; the amount of residual mobility in the atlanto-occipital and/or atlantoaxial joint; the presence of an extension deformity at an ankylosed C1–C2 area; and whether or not the C1/C2 segments are unstable. Is there is coronal imbalance of the trunk? Is there a flexion contracture in one of the hip joints?

▶ **Specific disclosures for patient consent.** Risk of paraplegia from mechanical compression or traction on the spinal cord during realignment. Paralysis due to vascular insufficiencies related to correction. Permanent or temporary radicular dysfunction. Postoperative hemorrhage. Infection. Loss of correction with risk of reoperation. Need for intraoperative wake-up test. Spinal cord monitoring.

Pedicle subtraction osteotomy is technically easier and particularly suitable for the lumbar spine. However, due to its anterior center of rotation, there is less correction in relation to the width of the osteotomy. In cases of osteoporosis there is a higher risk of loss of correction and implant failure.

Posterior open or minimally invasive osteotomy/instrumentation in combination with thoracoscopic anterior osteotomy/fusion is technically more difficult and surgically more demanding. In turn, the center of rotation as well as the amount of correction can be more accurately controlled and postoperative stability improved. Advantage: more safety with regard to surgically related neurological injuries. Disadvantage: additional anterior procedure.

Posterior open versus posterior minimally invasive procedure: intraoperative blood loss is significantly higher in an open procedure. Lengthy detachment of muscle is necessary, leading to a higher risk of postoperative wound infection (see below).

Disadvantages of the posterior minimally invasive osteotomy and stabilization: significantly prolonged duration of surgery and greater demands on operating room infrastructure.

Hemothorax, pneumothorax, or chylothorax as a complication of the transthoracic procedure and possible need for chest tube postoperatively should be discussed. Other possible complications the patient should be informed about are nerve root irritation/palsy, implant avulsion/breakage, injury to the thoracic or adjacent abdominal organs, retrograde ejaculation. In addition, damage to skin and cervical plexus related to positioning and unavoidable intraoperative changes of position are to be mentioned.

▶ Instruments

▶ **Posterior.** Pedicle screw-rod system with polyaxial heads.

When minimally invasive technique is applied: Percutaneous screw-rod system, favorable with in situ completable screws (Medicon). Basic spine tray with Kerrisons, chisels and rongeurs. Mono- and bipolar electrocautery. Surgical microscope with a minimum focus of 40 cm. Intraoperative radiography or navigation.

▶ **Anterior.** Set for thoracoscopically assisted procedures in prone position (Medicon). Interbody implants. 10-mm thoracoscope with video chain.

▶ **Anesthesia specifics.** Fiberoptic or video-assisted laryngoscopy intubation. Controlled hypotension. Anesthetic management must allow for spinal cord monitoring (sensory evoked potentials, better motor evoked potentials) and if necessary intraoperative wake-up test. A double-lumen endotracheal tube for one lung ventilation is normally not necessary, but the ability to do jet ventilation is desirable. Have 4 units of blood available for a posterior open procedure. If possible, the blood should be autologous and drawn preoperatively.

▶ **Position.** Prone on a spine table (segmentally adjustable so as to accommodate the initial kyphosis and the resulting correction). Headrest in a special cradle with a mirror to protect the eyes and nose as well as prevent pressure sores on the face. See ▶ Fig. 9.17.

▶ Approaches

▶ **Posterior.** For a conventional open procedure make a midline longitudinal incision depending on the instrumented area, usually from midthoracic to sacrum. Perform subperiosteal dissection bilaterally, including exposure of the joints and the bases of the transverse processes.

Posterior minimally invasive: Make transverse 15-mm stab incisions for each pedicle screw and a 3-cm midline skin incision for each osteotomy.

▶ **Anterior.** Two-portal technique for thoracoscopic osteotomy and fusion in the prone position:

1. Perform a 25-mm-long minithoracotomy parallel to the ribs on the lateral chest wall. This is placed at the junction of the posterior axillary line and the intervertebral disk space that will be osteotomized.
2. Make a 13-mm stab incision for the optical portal 20 mm farther proximal along the same intercostal space as the surgical incision (see ▶ Fig. 9.20).

▶ Minimally invasive surgical technique

▶ **Posterior screw implantation.** See ▶ Fig. 9.18.

▶ **Posterior minimally invasive osteotomy.** See ▶ Fig. 9.19.

▶ **Alternative: Pedicle subtraction osteotomy (PSO).** Many surgeons favor pedicle subtraction osteotomy because it avoids an additional anterior intervention. It is conventionally done in combination with open implantation of the anchoring screws, but it can also be performed with percutaneous screw implantation in a less invasive fashion. Since the surgical steps of PSO are identical, the latter is depicted here: As in ▶ Fig. 9.19e–h the osteotomy is placed approximately 1 cm caudal to the interspace and both pedicles are exposed. Perform either a subtotal (for example, cranial portion only) or total resection of the lamina including the spinous process and the pedicles. Finally, transversely resect or indent approximately 10 mm of the posterior wall. If the foramen is narrow preoperatively, a partial pedicle subtraction without intervention on the posterior wall is well suited to prevent a postcorrection foraminal stenosis. An anterior osteotomy can be avoided by performing a full PSO, but this comes at the cost of destabilization of the anterior column. Thus, this procedure is not indicated if osteoporosis is present. In addition, a PSO yields a smaller degree of correction per height of posterior osteotomy than does a back and front osteotomy due to the anteriorly located center of rotation for the correction. A more effective combination, therefore, is a posterior V-shaped osteotomy plus an anterior osteotomy.

▶ **Thoracoscopic anterior osteotomy.** See ▶ Fig. 9.20, ▶ Fig. 9.21.

▶ **Realignment.** See ▶ Fig. 9.22.

▶ **Posterior rod implantation.** See ▶ Fig. 9.23.

▶ **Filling the anterior defect, cage-assisted spondylodesis.** See ▶ Fig. 9.24.

▶ **Specific complications.** Injury to the dura. Neurologic deficits. Dislocation at the osteotomy site. Position-dependent pressure sores, particularly in nonsteroidal antirheumatic agent (NSAR)-induced malnutrition.

▶ **Postoperative aftercare.** Chest tube drainage for 2 days. Postoperative pain management. Respiratory exercise. Mobilization on the first postoperative day. No orthesis. No restrictions on sitting.

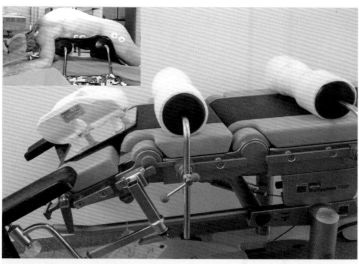

Fig. 9.17 Operating table for corrective surgery in the prone position; chest and pelvic supports to prevent compression of the abdominal organs; head cradle with mirror. The patient should be positioned to accommodate the preoperative postural malposition and to allow for intraoperative realignment. Unrestricted fluoroscopy of the thoracic and lumbar spine is possible in two planes.

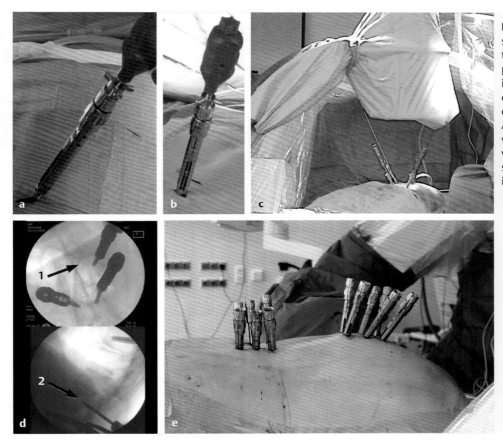

Fig. 9.18 Percutaneous insertion of the pedicle screws in T7, T8, and T9 as well as T12 and L1 through L3. **(a)** A screw is inserted down to the posterior spine through a transverse stab incision. **(b,c)** Aided by fluoroscopy the direction of the screw tip is oriented toward the pedicle entry point. **(d)** The medial pedicle wall (1 in the AP view) must only be crossed after the lateral view shows that the posterior edge of the vertebrae (2) has been reached. **(e)** All the screws and their head extenders have been implanted except L3.

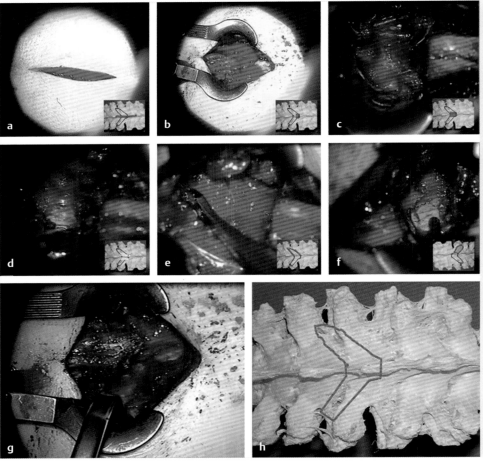

Fig. 9.19 V-Shaped minimally invasive Zielke's osteotomy technique, between T12 and L1. **(a)** Midline skin incision. **(b)** Resection of the ossified interspinous ligament. **(c)** Subtotal resection of the T12 spinous process and lamina. **(d)** The ligamentum flavum (yellow on model) is not ossified and lies exposed. **(e)** Osteotomy of the fused T12/L1 joint on the right is performed with a chisel. **(f)** View from the patient's right side: dura completely free in the mid portion. The osteotomy of the left joint is under way. **(g)** Overview again from the patient's left side showing the completed V-shaped osteotomy. **(h)** Photograph of the relevant posterior aspect of an ankylosing spondylitic spine. The osteotomy surfaces are shown in red (cranial is on the left).

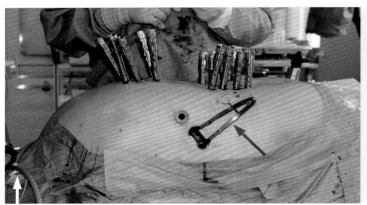

Fig. 9.20 Two-portal approach to the thoracic spine in the prone position. All of the posterior screws have been implanted, and the screw head extenders project from the stab incisions in the skin. A posterior V-shaped osteotomy is performed. Correction is not possible due to the ossification of the associated intervertebral disk. Therefore, a thoracoscopically assisted anterior osteotomy is performed through a two-portal approach. Portal 1: intercostal space dilated parallel to intact ribs using a spreader (arrow). Portal 2: same intercostal space, more proximal (green) for the endoscope.

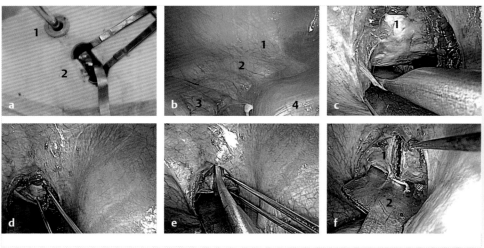

Fig. 9.21 **(a)** Delineation of the anterior approach with a thoracoscope (1) and working channel (2). **(b)** View through the thoracoscope of the surgical field at the thoracolumbar junction with spine (1), aorta (2), collapsed lung (3), and diaphragm (4). **(c)** The osteotomy site (1) between the twelfth thoracic and first lumbar vertebra has been dissected free. The aorta and paravertebral structures are secured with a metal retractor. **(d)** Two threaded-tip K-wires are inserted. They allow for fluoroscopic confirmation of positioning and help in guiding the chisel. **(e)** Osteotomy with a 20-mm chisel. **(f)** The osteotomy (1) has been performed but not yet opened. A metal retractor (2) protects the aorta.

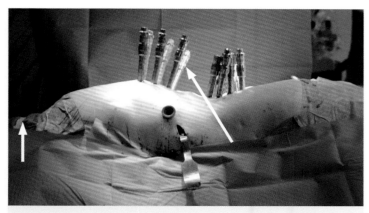

Fig. 9.22 After completion of the posterior and anterior osteotomies, correction is carried out by deflecting the table. Optimally, the rotational center of the spine lies just behind the posterior wall. This allows for the largest possible correction via closure of the posterior and opening of the anterior osteotomy. By comparing the head and neck region and the screw extensions (white arrows) in ▶ Fig. 9.20, the amount of correction becomes obvious.

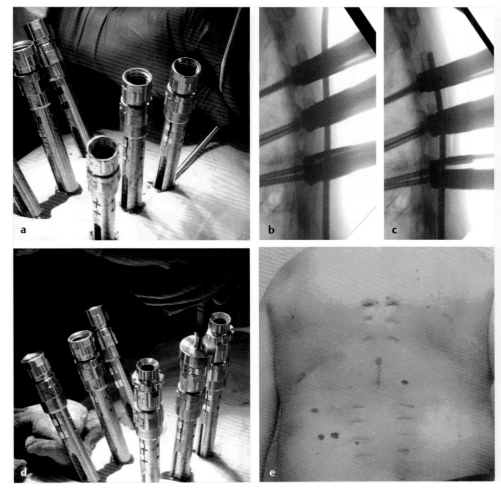

Fig. 9.23 (a) The 5.5-mm titanium rods are inserted into the screw extenders via the uppermost stab incision. **(b,c)** Lateral fluoroscopic images of a partially **(b)** and fully **(c)** inserted rod. **(d)** Fixation of the rod–screw connection at T8 through the screw extender. **(e)** All incisions delineated as postoperative scars.

9

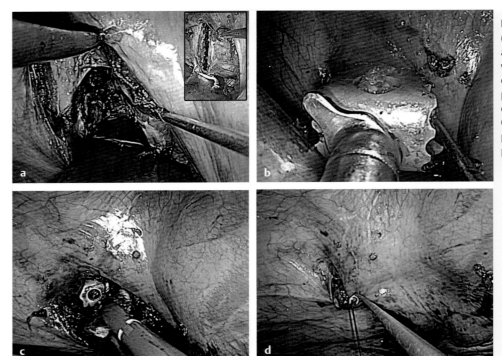

Fig. 9.24 (a) The osteotomy that in ▶ Fig. 9.21 (see small inset) had parallel edges is now angulated wide open. (b) A titanium cage filled with autologous bone (from the posterior osteotomy) is inserted. (c) The cage in its final position. Any remaining open space in the osteotomy is filled with cancellous bone. (d) Coverage of the implant through closure of the pleura via single sutures performed with a knot pusher.

9.3 Vertebral Body Augmentation through Vertebroplasty or Kyphoplasty

▶ **Indication.** Vertebral compression fracture(s) due to osteoporosis, including steroid induced, with continued substantial pain despite several weeks of conservative treatment. Progressive sintering with pathological kyphosis with little or moderate pain.

▶ **Pretherapeutic considerations.** Size of the defect: Is there a difference when comparing the lateral standing radiograph with the sagittal MRI scan? Location of the defect: How near is it to the disk space, to draining veins or fractures at the end plate or posterior wall? Depending on these factors select cement viscosity and choose between vertebroplasty and kyphoplasty. It must also be decided whether to perform a uniportal or bilateral procedure and afterward whether to use general anesthesia or analgesic sedation.

▶ **Specific disclosures for patient consent.** Extravasation. Benefits and risks of kyphoplasty vs. vertebroplasty. Quantity of cement. Risk of fractures in other vertebrae or continued sintering with painfully increasing kyphosis. Risk of vertebral body necrosis and postinterventional infection (ranging from locally manageable to requiring a corpectomy).

▶ **Instruments.** Basic vertebroplasty and kyphoplasty instrument sets. Standard frame for spine procedures in prone position that prevents pressure on the abdomen and allows gravitational correction of kyphosis. Radiolucent operating table; image intensifier, preferably with a double monitor; ideally a second imager, one for each plane. Clock with second hand.

▶ **Position.** See ▶ Fig. 9.25.

▶ **Intraoperative fluoroscopy.** In principle, one radiologic image intensifier is sufficient for cannula insertion. Start with AP view and direct the beam exactly parallel to the upper end plate of the target vertebra. The tip of the cannula should project onto the craniolateral edge of the pedicle, and remain lateral to the medial pedicle edge after advancing 15 mm. The C-arm should be swung 90° into the lateral view before proceeding any further.

This requires time and partial sterile redraping after every swing of the C-arm. See ▶ Fig. 9.26. If possible, two machines with sterile draping should be used because cement injection is considerably safer while imaging in both planes. A right-handed surgeon is positioned on the left side of the patient and the surgical nurse at the foot end.

▶ **Surgical technique.** See ▶ Fig. 9.27, ▶ Fig. 9.28, ▶ Fig. 9.29, ▶ Fig. 9.30, ▶ Fig. 9.31, ▶ Fig. 9.32, ▶ Fig. 9.33. The decision between vertebroplasty and kyphoplasty depends upon the fracture realignment obtained by prone positioning and manual extension. The example here shows T11 and T12 vertebroplasties and an L2 kyphoplasty for a case with fractures of both end plates and a central impression of the body: Since this situation carries the risk of inadequate correction and extravasation of the cement into a disk space, we decided against balloon kyphoplasty in favor of a mesh to contain and channel the injected cement.

▶ **Specific complications.** Injury to neural or paravertebral structures resulting from incorrect cannula placement. Extravasation in the disk space, the vascular system, or the spinal canal. Allergic reaction to cement application. Emboli in the vascular systems of heart and lungs with cardiac or pulmonary sequelae.

▶ **Postoperative aftercare.** Mobilization, full weight bearing, and isometric exercises are allowed after 4 hours. Review and optimize management of rheumatoid/osteoporosis medication.

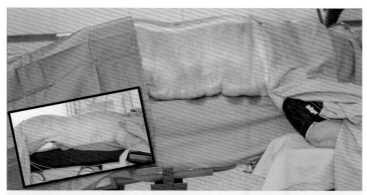

Fig. 9.25 A patient prone on a spine frame with bolsters in the groin area. The arms are placed on arm holders lined with gel pads (small inset). This allows fluoroscopic imaging in both AP and lateral orientations.

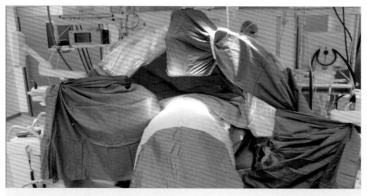

Fig. 9.26 Two image intensifiers are arranged in such a way that fluoroscopy can be performed in two planes.

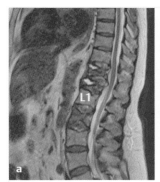
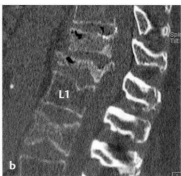
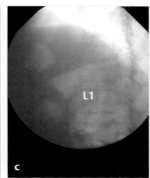

Fig. 9.27 (a) Preoperative MRI. (b) CT scan shows recent end plate impressions at T11 and T12 and an old fracture at the T12 posterior wall. Osteoporotic indentations of the upper and lower endplates of L2 are seen. (c) Intra-operative fluoroscopy image after induction of anesthesia and muscle relaxation. Prone positioning alone has partially corrected T12 when compared to the preoperative CT and MRI. However, the height of L2 is even less than it was in (a) and (b).

Therapeutic decision: Vertebroplasty is performed at T11 and T12. However, at L2, a kyphoplasty will facilitate straightening and prevent the risk of extravasation into the L2 disk space. High-viscosity cement is used because the augmentation will be performed in the immediate vicinity of the end plate.

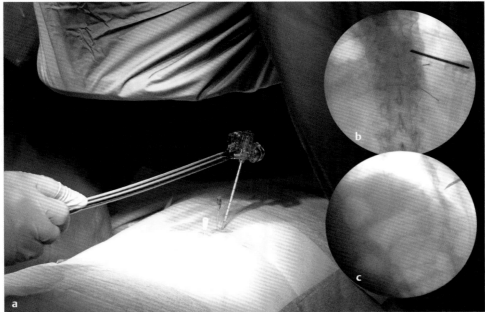

Fig. 9.28 Starting point of the cannula depicted in precise AP and lateral fluoroscopic views. (a) The cannula is advanced until contact is made with bone. (b) A corresponding fluoroscopic AP image of the tip and the upper lateral aspect of the pedicle. (c) A lateral image to verify the correct cranial/caudal entrance point.

9

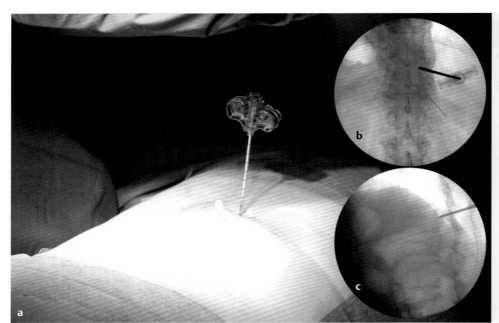

Fig. 9.29 (a–c) The cannula is advanced safely past the spinal canal before entering the vertebral body. When using bevel edged cannula tips, a slight change in direction can be achieved merely by rotation.

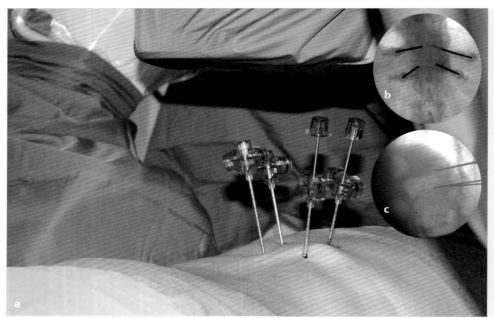

Fig. 9.30 (a–c) All cannulas have been inserted for a biportal vertebroplasty. Partially withdrawing the obturator on one side helps to differentiate right from left in the lateral view.

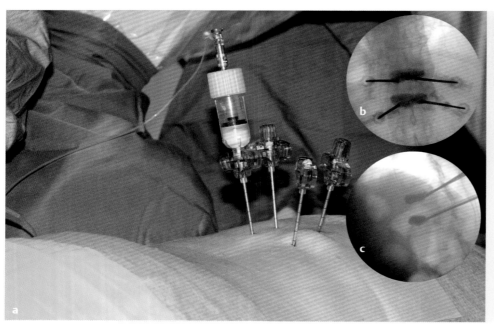

Fig. 9.31 (a–c) Cement application at T11 and T12 without extravasation. Cannulas remain in place until the cement has hardened. They are rotated occasionally to prevent them from becoming fixed.

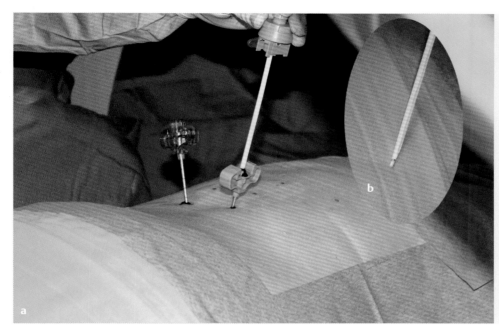

Fig. 9.32 (a) A right-sided large-caliber cannula is inserted into L2 using the same technique. **(b)** The tip of the mesh with radiographic markings.

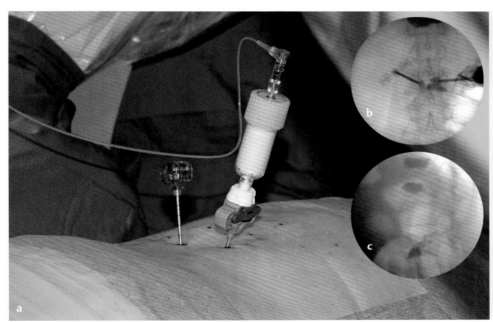

Fig. 9.33 Cement injection in L2. The cement reaches the cranial and caudal end plates with no extravasation. A comparison with ▶ Fig. 9.27c shows that the vertebral body has reached almost its original height.

9

Index